Preface

This book is intended as an aid to oral medicine and the diagnosis and treatment of oral disease. The format chosen has been to describe diseases initially by site, as this is how patients present: inevitably this leads to some overlap. Because of its increasing importance, HIV disease is given a separate section.

The text and illustrations cover the common conditions seen in oral medicine, and some of the less common and exotic. It cannot be fully comprehensive, particularly since not all of oral medicine lends itself to illustrative presentation—too many patients have symptoms but no signs of disease; and because of space. For reasons of space, pictures of oral and perioral lesions only have been included. Nevertheless, we have covered a wide range of material and trust that this together with the treatment synopses will be useful to undergraduates, postgraduates and practitioners.

A few illustrations show ungloved fingers. These are usually not the clinician's fingers. Protective gloves should always be worn by clinicians.

London, 1999

C. S.
R. A. C.

Contents

Herpes labialis

Incidence/ Aetiology

Common, especially in immunocompromised. Herpes simplex virus (HSV), usually type 1. HSV latent in trigeminal ganglion is reactivated as herpes labialis ('cold sores'). Precipitated by sun, fever, trauma, menstruation, HIV disease, immunosuppression, etc.

Clinical features

Prodromal paraesthesia or irritation. Erythema, then vesicles at/near mucocutaneous junction of lip. Heals in 7–10 days (Figs 1 & 2).

Investigations/ Diagnosis

Viral damage can be confirmed by smear. Differentiate from zoster, impetigo, or carcinoma (rarely).

Treatment

Penciclovir or aciclovir cream applied in prodrome. Immunocompromised may need systemic aciclovir (oral or i.v.).

Herpes zoster ('shingles')

Incidence/ Aetiology

Mainly affects elderly, or immunocompromised, such as in HIV infection. Varicella-zoster virus (VZV), latent in sensory ganglion (see also p. 31). Reactivated often by immunosuppression.

Clinical features

Pain and rash in trigeminal dermatome (Fig. 3). Unilateral vesicles, then mouth ulcers. Potentially lethal in HIV infection.

Investigations/ Diagnosis

Clinical features. Smears show viral damaged cells. Pain: may simulate toothache. Rash: differentiate from HSV infection. Mouth ulcers (see p. 23).

Treatment

Analgesics. Aciclovir cream to rash, and tablets; intravenous aciclovir for immunocompromised.

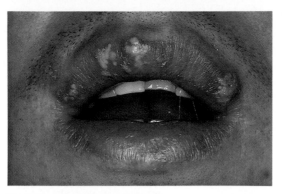

Fig. 1 Herpes labialis: vesicular stage.

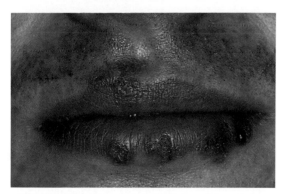

Fig. 2 Herpes labialis: later, crusting stage.

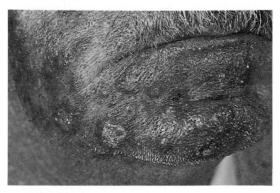

Fig. 3 Herpes zoster: intact vesicles and crusted lesions on lip and chin.

Impetigo contagiosa

Incidence/
Aetiology

Uncommon: mainly in underprivileged children (2–6 years). Highly contagious. Usually Streptococci (group A). *Staphylococcus aureus* phage type 71 causes *bullous impetigo*, a severe form with fever ± toxic epidermal necrolysis.

Clinical features

Papules then vesicles surrounded by erythema then multiple pustules with golden crust (Fig. 4). Regional lymphadenitis sometimes, but systemic symptoms rare. Lesions spread by touch to other areas.

Investigations/
Diagnosis

Culture of pus. Differentiate from other vesiculo-bullous diseases. On lips, herpes labialis is the prime differential diagnosis.

Treatment

No systemic illness: chlortetracycline cream. Systemic symptoms: oral flucloxacillin.

Primary syphilis (Hunterian or hard chancre)

Incidence/
Aetiology

Rare on lip (upper) or intraorally—usually tongue. Primary infection with *Treponema pallidum* (see also p. 39).

Clinical features

Small papule develops into large painless indurated ulcer (Fig. 5), with regional lymphadenitis. Chancre heals spontaneously in 1–2 months.

Investigations/
Diagnosis

T. pallidum in smear (darkfield examination). Serology positive late in this stage. Differentiate from trauma, herpes labialis, pyogenic granuloma, carcinoma. Very rarely: non-venereal treponematoses.

Treatment

Penicillin (depot injection); if allergic to penicillin, use erythromycin or tetracycline.

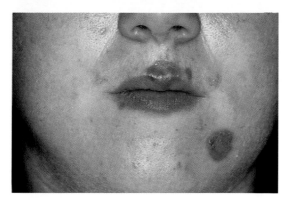

Fig. 4 Impetigo contagiosa.

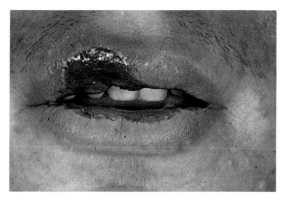

Fig. 5 Syphilis: primary chancre on upper lip.

Pyogenic granuloma

Incidence/
Aetiology

Uncommon. Possibly reactive vascular lesion. Inflammatory infiltrate is superimposed. Intraoral lesions sometimes associated with pregnancy.

Clinical features

Small (<3 cm) red painless mass. Bleeds easily, ulcerates and grows rapidly (Fig. 6). Frequently seen on gingival margin, tongue, or rarely the lip. Unlikely to resolve without treatment.

Investigations/
Diagnosis

Histopathology. Differentiate from angiomatous proliferations, chancre, carcinoma, Kaposi's sarcoma.

Treatment

Excision.

Carcinoma

Incidence/
Aetiology

Uncommon in developed countries. Elderly males predominate. Predisposing factors include UV irradiation (sun), immunosuppression, tobacco, carcinogens and coal tar derivatives (see also pp. 45 & 69).

Clinical features

Thickening, induration, crusting or ulceration, usually at vermilion border of lower lip just to one side of midline (Figs 7 & 8). Late involvement of the submental lymph nodes.

Investigations/
Diagnosis

Biopsy is confirmatory. Differentiate from herpes labialis, keratoacanthoma, and (rarely) basal cell carcinoma (on skin), molluscum contagiosum.

Treatment

Wedge resection or irradiation. (The prognosis is good: 70% 5-year survival.)

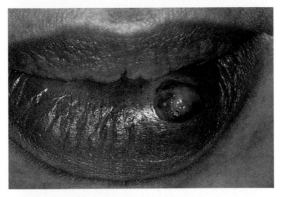

Fig. 6 Pyogenic granuloma.

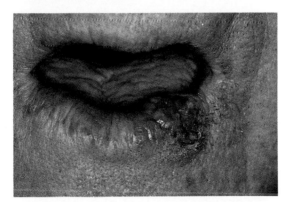

Fig. 7 Carcinoma of lower lip in elderly male in common site.

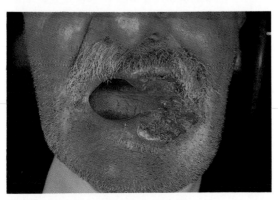

Fig. 8 Advanced carcinoma involving both lips.

Erythema multiforme

Incidence/ Aetiology

Uncommon. Mainly young adult males. Putative reactions to microorganisms (herpes simplex, mycoplasma), to drugs (e.g. sulphonamides) or to other factors.

Clinical features

May affect mouth alone, or skin and/or other mucosae. The minor form affects only one site. The major form (Stevens–Johnson syndrome) is widespread, with fever and toxicity. Mouth: serosanguinous exudate on ulcerated swollen lips, and ulcers (Figs 9 & 10). Rashes: various but typically 'target' lesions or bullae.

Investigations/ Diagnosis

Clinical picture; biopsy sometimes helpful. Differentiate from other lip lesions, and other causes of mouth ulcers (see p. 23).

Treatment

Minor form: symptomatic treatment $\pm$ aciclovir. Major form: systemic corticosteroids and/or azathioprine or other immunomodulatory drugs.

Leukaemia

Incidence/ Aetiology

Uncommon: 50–60% leukaemias are acute. Acute lymphocytic leukaemia affects mainly children; acute myeloid leukaemia affects mainly young adults; chronic myeloid leukaemia seen mainly in middle-aged adults; chronic lymphocytic leukaemia seen mainly in the elderly. Ionizing radiation, immunosuppression, chemicals, chromosomal disorders (see also pp. 43 & 127).

Clinical features

Recurrent labial and intraoral herpes virus infections (see p. 1); purpura with bleeding into lesions; leukaemic deposits (Fig. 11; see p. 43).

Investigations/ Diagnosis

Blood picture and marrow biopsy. Differentiate from herpes labialis and erythema multiforme.

Treatment

Cytotoxic chemotherapy of leukaemia; treat herpes labialis (see p. 1).

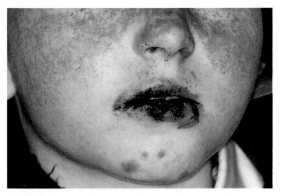

Fig. 9 Erythema multiforme: crusting bloodstained lesions.

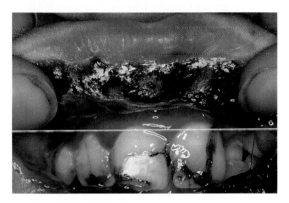

Fig. 10 Erythema multiforme: ulceration of the lips.

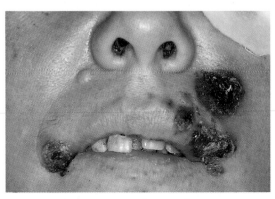

Fig. 11 Acute leukaemia: ulceration of leukaemic deposits.

Discoid lupus erythematosus (DLE)

Incidence/
Aetiology

Rare: usually in females. Oral lesions in up to 25% of those with cutaneous DLE. Drugs, hormones and viruses may contribute in genetically predisposed persons (see also p. 55).

Clinical features

Mainly affects buccal mucosa, gingiva and lip. Lesions on vermilion border are scaly and crusting (Fig. 12) (intraoral lesions, see p. 55).

Investigations/
Diagnosis

Biopsy; serology sometimes informative. Differentiate from systemic lupus erythematosus, lichen planus, leukoplakia (keratosis), and carcinoma.

Treatment

Topical corticosteroids; cryosurgery or excision of localised lesions. Small predisposition to carcinoma.

Lichen planus

Incidence/
Aetiology

Lichen planus rarely involves lips or facial skin. Mainly a disease of middle-aged/elderly females (see also pp. 55 & 57). Unclear aetiology.

Clinical features

White striae (Fig. 13), rarely papular lesions or plaque, or atrophic or erosive lesions on lips.

Investigations/
Diagnosis

Biopsy, but findings may be inconclusive. Differentiate from lupus erythematosus, leukoplakia (keratosis), chronic candidosis and carcinoma.

Treatment

Topical corticosteroids.

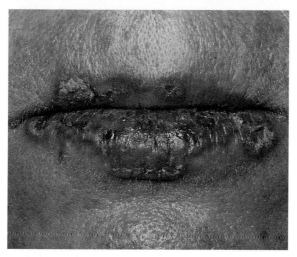

Fig. 12 Discoid lupus erythematosus: erythematous and scaling lesions on vermilion border of lip.

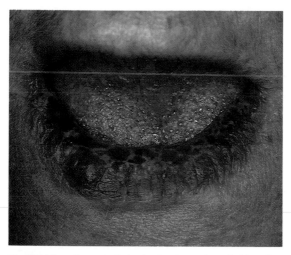

Fig. 13 Lichen planus: typical striae (angioma also coincidentally present).

Angular stomatitis (angular cheilitis)

Incidence/ Aetiology

Common, mainly elderly edentulous patients. Usually due to *Candida albicans. Staph. aureus* and/or streptococci may also be cultured. Most patients have denture-induced stomatitis (see p. 77). Other causes include iron deficiency, hypovitaminoses (especially B), malabsorption states (e.g. Crohn's disease), HIV infection and other immune defects.

Clinical features

Symmetrical erythematous fissures on skin of commissures (Figs 14 & 15), and (rarely) commissural leukoplakia intraorally.

Investigations/ Diagnosis

Clinical features diagnostic: blood picture; smears for fungal hyphae.

Treatment

Eliminate any underlying systemic predisposing factors. Treat denture-induced stomatitis (see p. 77). If angular stomatitis persists, treat with topical antifungal such as miconazole.

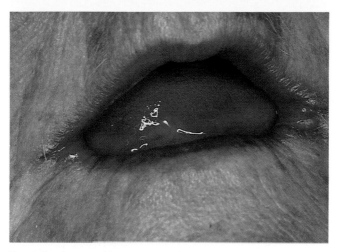

Fig. 14 Angular stomatitis secondary to denture-induced stomatitis.

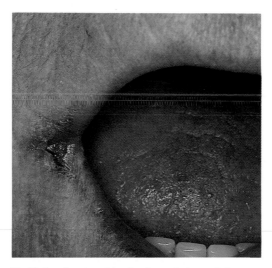

Fig. 15 Angular stomatitis: showing typical spread along natural fissure.

Cracked lip

Incidence/ Aetiology

Common during cold, windy, winter weather. Chronic (self-induced) trauma and maceration, and mouth breathing. Also found in Crohn's disease and Down syndrome.

Clinical features

Usually single persistent painful vertical fissure which bleeds on stretching the lip and opening the mouth wide (Fig. 16).

Investigations/ Diagnosis

Clinical features diagnostic. Differentiate from angular stomatitis (occasionally).

Treatment

Bland creams (Boots E45); rarely excision (curative).

Actinic burns

Incidence/ Aetiology

Mainly in fair-skinned individuals in sunny climes or at high altitude. Shortwave UV light (sunlight may also trigger herpes labialis and lupus erythematosus).

Clinical features

Erythema, oedema, vesiculation and occasionally haemorrhage (Fig. 17); later whitish lesion or keratosis.

Investigations/ Diagnosis

History and clinical features; biopsy may help. Differentiate from other causes of burns (e.g. friction and heat).

Treatment

Prophylaxis: bland or barrier creams (Uvistat).

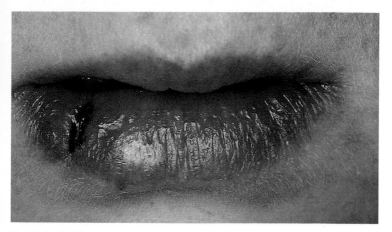

Fig. 16 Cracked lip.

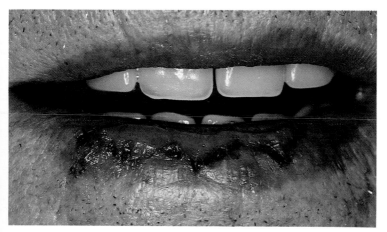

Fig. 17 Actinic cheilitis: typically affects lower lip, as here.

Allergic angioedema

Incidence/ Aetiology

Uncommon: mainly in those with atopic tendency. Type 1 allergic response to allergen.

Clinical features

Rapid development of oedematous swelling of lip(s). Oedema may involve neck and hazard the airway (Fig. 18).

Investigations/ Diagnosis

History of atopic disease and/or exposure to allergen; allergy testing. Differentiate from hereditary angioedema and other causes of diffuse facial swelling including: oedema from trauma, infection or insect bite; surgical emphysema; Crohn's disease, cheilitis granulomatosa and Melkersson–Rosenthal syndrome; cheilitis glandularis; lymphangioma; haemangioma.

Treatment

Mild angioedema: antihistamines.
Severe angioedema: intramuscular adrenaline, and i.v. corticosteroids.

Hereditary angioedema

Incidence/ Aetiology

Rare genetic defect of inhibitor of activated first component of complement C1 (C1 esterase inhibitor); autosomal dominant inheritance.

Clinical features

As in allergic angioedema (above) but precipitated by trauma, e.g. dental treatment. High mortality in some families.

Investigations/ Diagnosis

Family history. C1 esterase inhibitor and C4 serum levels are low. Differentiate from acute allergic angioedema and other causes of facial swelling.

Treatment

Stanozolol (an androgenic steroid).

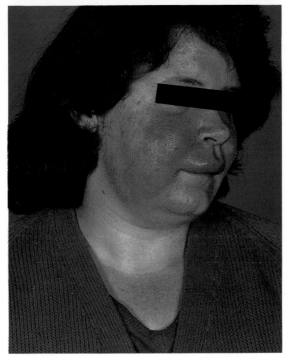

Fig. 18 Acute angioedema: acute and hereditary types are clinically indistinguishable.

Oral Crohn's disease

Incidence/ Aetiology

Uncommon but increasing. Mainly young adults. Unknown aetiology.

Clinical features

Facial and/or labial swelling (Fig. 19); angular stomatitis and/or cracked lips; ulcers, mucosal tags and/or cobble-stoning (see Figs 112 & 113, p. 104); gingival hyperplasia. Sometimes effects of malabsorption (see pp. 11, 23 & 115). Miescher's cheilitis is where lip swelling is seen in isolation. Melkersson–Rosenthal syndrome is facial swelling with fissured tongue and facial palsy.

Investigations/ Diagnosis

Differentiate from orofacial granulomatosis (p. 47) sarcoid, tuberculosis and foreign body reactions by gastrointestinal investigation or symptoms.

Treatment

Intralesional corticosteroids; occasionally sulphasalazine; eliminate food allergens.

Sarcoidosis

Incidence/ Aetiology

Uncommon: prevalence highest in black females. Unknown aetiology: chronic granulomatous reaction.

Clinical features

Cervical lymphadenopathy; enlarged salivary glands and xerostomia (see Fig. 153, p. 138); mucosal nodules; gingival hyperplasia; labial swelling (Fig. 20); rarely, Heerfordt syndrome (salivary and lacrimal swelling, facial palsy and uveitis).

Investigations/ Diagnosis

Biopsy; chest radiograph; gallium scan; raised serum angiotensin converting enzyme and adenosine deaminase. Differentiate from Crohn's disease, tuberculosis and foreign body reactions.

Treatment

Intralesional corticosteroids; systemic steroids if lung or eye involved.

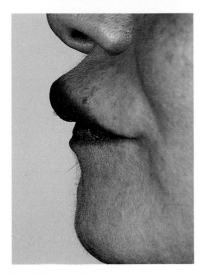

Fig. 19 Crohn's disease: persistent macrocheilia.

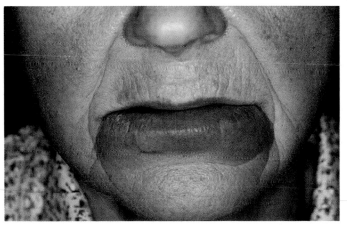

Fig. 20 Sarcoidosis: note clinical similarity to Figure 19.

Naevi

Incidence/ Aetiology

Rare. Usually affect lips, palate, gingiva, or buccal mucosa. Congenital lesions of proliferating melanocytes (see also p. 87).

Clinical features

Usually asymptomatic smooth pigmented macule < 1 cm in diameter (Fig. 21).

Investigations/ Diagnosis

A biopsy, showing naevus cells, is essential to exclude malignant melanoma. Differentiate from racial pigmentation, amalgam tattoo, malignant melanoma and Peutz–Jeghers syndrome (see p. 81).

Treatment

Excision biopsy.

Peutz–Jeghers syndrome

Incidence/ Aetiology

Rare. Autosomal dominant disorder (see also p. 83).

Clinical features

Pigmented macules periorally and on labial and/or buccal mucosa (Fig. 22), rarely on trunk or extremities. Gastrointestinal polyps—usually benign and in small intestine, predisposing to intussusception.

Investigations/ Diagnosis

Clinical features pathognomonic. Differentiate from racial pigmentation and freckles (ephelides) (see p. 81).

Treatment

Reassure or excise for histological confirmation.

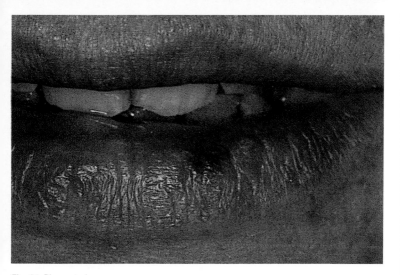

Fig. 21 Pigmented naevus.

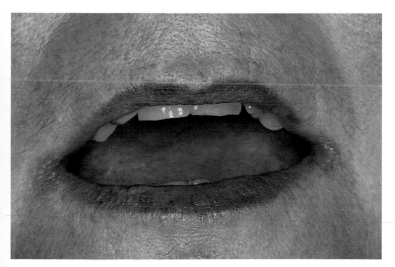

Fig. 22 Peutz–Jeghers syndrome: multiple pigmented macules.

Mucocele

Incidence/ Aetiology

Common: mostly on lower lip and in young adults/children, particularly males. It sometimes affects tongue, buccal mucosa or floor of mouth. Usually extravasation of mucus from damaged salivary gland duct; rarely retention of mucus within a salivary gland or duct (see also p. 101).

Clinical features

Dome-shaped, bluish, translucent, fluctuant painless swellings, usually ⩽ 1 cm in diameter (Fig. 23). These rupture easily to release viscid salty mucus, but frequently recur.

Investigations/ Diagnosis

Microscopic features. Diagnosis is clearcut but a salivary gland neoplasm must be excluded, particularly in cystic swellings in *upper* lip.

Treatment

If asymptomatic and small, observe; otherwise, use cryosurgery or excision including associated gland.

Sturge–Weber syndrome (encephalotrigeminal angiomatosis)

Incidence/ Aetiology

Rare congenital angioma (hamartoma) that affects face, mouth and ipsilateral leptomeninges (see also p. 75).

Clinical features

Haemangioma (port-wine naevus) in trigeminal region involving face (naevus flammeus), oral mucosa (Fig. 24) and underlying bone (with hemihypertrophy of bone and accelerated eruption of associated teeth); epilepsy and intracerebral calcifications; gingival hyperplasia (often phenytoin-induced); mentally challenged.

Diagnosis

Differentiate from haemangioma and other rare syndromes.

Treatment

Anticonvulsants for epilepsy; observation of angioma, or treatment as for haemangioma (see p. 75).

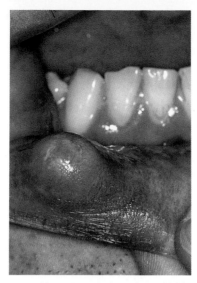

Fig. 23 Mucocele: typical translucent bluish appearance in the characteristic site.

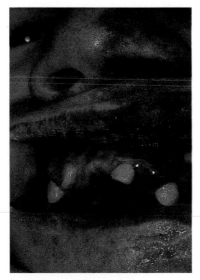

Fig. 24 Sturge–Weber syndrome: mucocutaneous angiomatosis stopping sharply at the midline.

Ulcers of local aetiology

Incidence/ Aetiology

Common. Trauma, including self-induced lesions due to cheek biting (a neurotic habit) and in some rare syndromes (Figs 25 & 26). Orthodontic appliances, dentures, or interdental wiring are common iatrogenic causes. Other types include pterygoid ulcers of palate in neonates (Bednar's aphthae), and ulcers due to burns (from electrical injury, heat or cold, chemicals or irradiation). Rare causes include ulceration of lingual fraenum caused by repeated coughing.

Clinical features

Usually a single ulcer closely related to cause (e.g. denture flange). Chronic irritation may cause hyperplasia or hyperkeratosis.

Diagnosis

Differentiate from mouth ulcers which can be caused by:
- Malignant neoplasms
- Recurrent aphthae (and Behçet syndrome)
- Systemic disorders
    i. *Haematological*: haematinic (iron, folate, vitamin B_{12}) deficiency, white cell and other immune defects including HIV infection, and leukaemia.
    ii. *Gastrointestinal*: coeliac disease, Crohn's disease and ulcerative colitis.
    iii. *Mucocutaneous* (dermatological): lichen planus, pemphigus, pemphigoid (and localized oral purpura), erythema multiforme, dermatitis herpetiformis (and linear IgA disease), epidermolysis bullosa, lupus erythematosus and Reiter syndrome.
    iv. *Infections*: herpes viruses, Coxsackie viruses, syphilis, tuberculosis and deep mycoses.
    v. *Drugs*: cytotoxic agents and many others.

Treatment

Remove aetiological factors. Local treatment: chlorhexidine mouthwash.

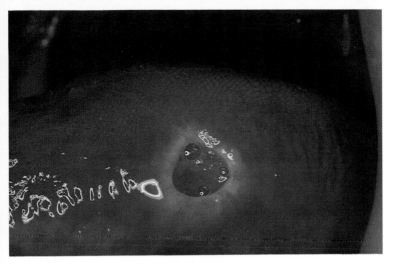

Fig. 25 Traumatic ulcer with rim of frictional keratosis.

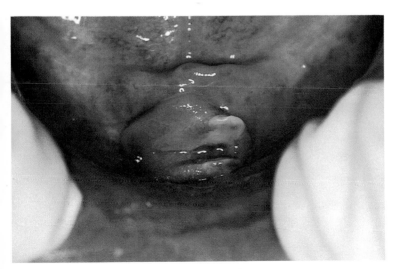

Fig. 26 Traumatic ulcer caused by denture flange.

Aphthae (recurrent aphthous stomatitis— RAS)

Incidence/ Aetiology

Unclear: immunological changes are detectable but there is no reliable evidence of autoimmune disease or any classical immunological reactions. They may be due to changes in cell-mediated immune responses and cross-reactivity with *Streptococcus sanguis*. Underlying predisposing factors are seen in a minority: haematinic (iron, folate or vitamin B_{12}) deficiency in *c.* 10%, relationship with luteal phase of menstruation (rarely), 'stress', food allergies (possibly) and HIV/AIDS (major aphthae).

C. 25% of population, mostly non-smokers. Onset is usually in childhood or adolescence. Later onset may signify haematinic deficiency or HIV/AIDS.

Clinical features

Typically: early onset with recurrent ulcers usually lasting 1 week to 1 month. There may be multiple oral ulcers; otherwise normal health. There are three distinct clinical patterns of aphthae:
- *Minor*—small ulcers (<4 mm) on mobile mucosae, healing within 14 days, no scarring (Fig. 27)
- *Major*—large ulcers (may >1 cm), any site including dorsum of tongue and hard palate, healing within 1–3 m, with scarring (Fig. 28)
- *Herpetiform ulcers*—multiple minute ulcers that coalesce to produce ragged ulcers (Fig. 29).

Investigations/ Diagnosis

History of recurrences and clinical features. There is no immunological test of value. A blood picture is useful for possible deficiencies (Fig. 30, p. 28). Differentiate from other causes of mouth ulcers (see p. 23), especially Behçet syndrome (p. 27).

Treatment

Treat any underlying predisposing factors. Treat aphthae with chlorhexidine mouthwash or topical corticosteroids or tetracycline rinses. Rarely, more potent topical steroids (e.g. betamethasone or beclomethasone) may be needed.

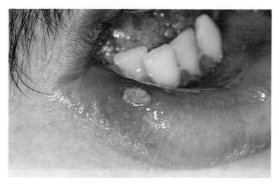

Fig. 27 Minor aphthae: typical ulcer with surrounding erythema.

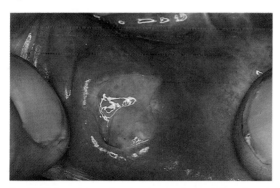

Fig. 28 Major aphthae: also showing scarring and distortion of mucosa.

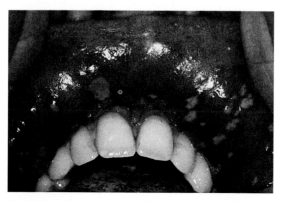

Fig. 29 Herpetiform aphthae: multiple ulcers have coalesced to form irregular lesions.

Behçet syndrome

Incidence/
Aetiology

Unclear: immunological changes like those in aphthae are reported. Immune complexes, possibly with herpes simplex virus, may be implicated in persons with specific HLA associations (HLA-B 5101).

Rare: most common in Japan and Turkey. Predominantly affects adult males.

Clinical features

Multi-system disorder in which oral lesions are indistinguishable from typical aphthae.
- *Oral aphthae*: almost invariably (Fig. 31).
- *Eye disease*: reduced visual acuity, uveitis, retinal vasculitis.
- *Skin disease*: typically erythema nodosum.
- *Joint disease*: arthralgia of large joints.
- *Neurological disease*: various syndromes.
- *Others*: thromboses, colitis, renal disease, etc.

Investigations/
Diagnosis

Clinical features. No immunological test of value. Differentiate from other oculomucocutaneous disorders, especially ulcerative colitis, erythema multiforme, syphilis and Reiter syndrome.

Treatment

- *Oral ulcers*: treat as for aphthae (above).
- *Systemic*: immunosuppression using colchicine, corticosteroids, azathioprine, cyclosporin, dapsone or thalidomide (not if there is any possibility of pregnancy).

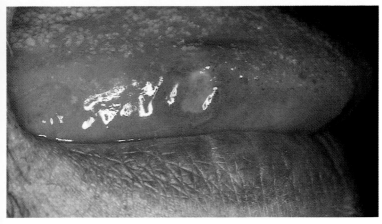

Fig 30 Minor aphthae secondary to vitamin B_{12} deficiency.

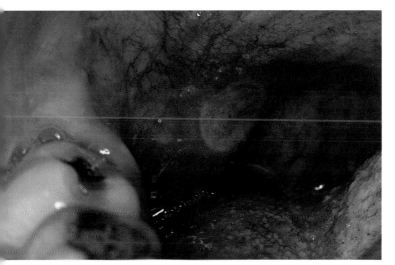

Fig. 31 Behçet syndrome: aphthae indistinguishable from 'simple' aphthae.

Herpetic stomatitis

Incidence/
Aetiology

Common cause of mouth ulcers, with fever in children. It is also seen in adults, especially in more affluent communities. Herpes simplex virus (HSV), usually type 1 (see also p. 131).

Clinical features

Incubation period 3–7 days. Some 50% of infections are subclinical. Clinical features of primary infection include:
- *Mouth ulcers*: multiple vesicles and round scattered ulcers (Figs 32 & 33) with yellow slough and erythematous halo; ulcers fuse to produce irregular lesions
- *Gingivitis*: diffuse erythema and oedema, occasionally haemorrhagic
- *Cervical lymphadenitis*
- *Fever*
- *Malaise, irritability* and *anorexia*
- *Rarely*: skin or eye involvement.
  Dental staff may acquire a herpetic whitlow if not wearing surgical gloves. Recurrences usually present as herpes labialis (see p. 1), and/or intraoral ulcers in immunocompromised (Fig. 34). Infection may rarely precipitate erythema multiforme.

Investigation/
Diagnosis

Smear for viral damaged cells. Viral culture, immunofluorescence or electron microscopy are used occasionally. A rising titre of antibodies is confirmatory. Differentiate from other causes of mouth ulcers (see p. 23), especially hand, foot and mouth disease, chickenpox, shingles, herpangina, erythema multiforme and leukaemia.

Treatment

Soft diet and adequate fluid intake; antipyretics/analgesics (paracetamol elixir); local antiseptics (0.2% aqueous chlorhexidine mouthwashes); aciclovir orally or parenterally in immunocompromised patients.

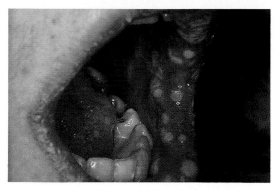

Fig. 32 Herpetic stomatitis: vesicles and ulcers extending to inner aspect of lower lip.

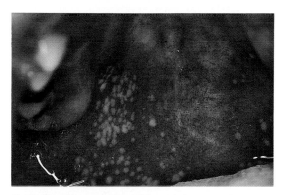

Fig. 33 Herpetic stomatitis: vesicles and ulcers on palate.

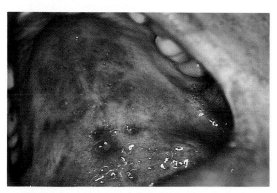

Fig. 34 Herpetic vesicles in palate of patient with HIV infection.

Chickenpox (varicella)

Incidence/ Aetiology	Herpes varicella-zoster virus (VZV); common childhood exanthem.
Clinical features	Incubation period 14–21 days. Some 50% of infections are subclinical. Clinical features include:

- *Ulcers*: indistinguishable from HSV, but no associated gingivitis (Fig. 35)
- *Rash*: mainly face and trunk; papules then vesicles, pustules and scabs, in crops
- *Cervical lymphadenitis*
- *Fever*
- *Malaise, irritability, anorexia*
- *Rarely*: pneumonia or encephalitis.

Investigations/ Diagnosis	Clinical diagnosis. Rising antibody titre is confirmatory. Differentiate from other mouth ulcers, especially herpes simplex and other viral infections (see p. 23).
Treatment	Symptomatic (see p. 29); immune globulin or aciclovir in immunocompromised.

Shingles (zoster)

Incidence/ Aetiology	Uncommon. Reactivation of VZV latent in sensory ganglia. Immune defects predispose to reactivation, usually in elderly.
Clinical features	

- *Majority thoracic*: 30% trigeminal region.
- *Pain*: before, with and after rash.
- *Rash*: unilateral vesiculating then scabbing in dermatome, in V_2 and/or V_3 area.
- *Mouth ulcers*: *mandibular zoster*—ipsilateral on buccal and lingual mucosa; *maxillary*—ipsilateral on palate and vestibule (Fig. 36).
- *Rarely*: geniculate zoster (rash in ear, facial palsy and ulcers on ipsilateral soft palate)—Ramsay–Hunt syndrome.

Investigations/ Diagnosis	Clinical diagnosis. Smear may help. Differentiate from toothache and other causes of ulcers, especially herpes simplex (see p. 23).
Treatment	Analgesics; aciclovir (high dose) orally or parenterally, especially in the immunocompromised; symptomatic treatment of ulcers. Ophthalmic zoster: ophthalmological opinion.

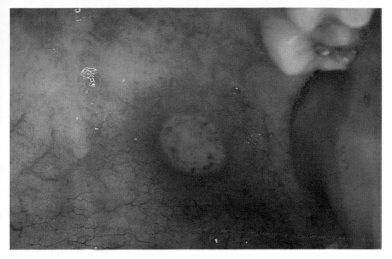

Fig. 35 Chickenpox.

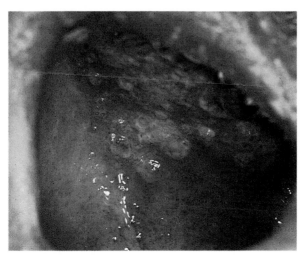

Fig. 36 Zoster: confluent vesiculation and ulceration of palate.

Hand-foot-and-mouth disease

Incidence/
Aetiology

Common. It usually causes small epidemics, in children, but is rarely seen in dental practice. Coxsackie A viruses (usually A16; rarely A5 or 10).

Clinical features

Incubation period 2–6 days. Infections may be subclinical. Clinical features include: oral ulcers, resembling herpetic stomatitis but affecting labial and buccal mucosa (Fig. 37); no gingivitis; mild fever, malaise and anorexia; rash—red papules that evolve to superficial vesicles in a few days, mainly on palms and soles.

Investigations/
Diagnosis

Clinical diagnosis. Serology is confirmatory but rarely required. Differentiate from herpetic stomatitis, chickenpox.

Treatment

Symptomatic (see herpes simplex, p. 29).

Herpangina

Incidence/
Aetiology

Uncommon. Small outbreaks are seen among young children. Coxsackie viruses usually (A7, 9, 16; B1, 2, 3, 4, or 5); echoviruses (9 or 17).

Clinical features

Incubation period 2–9 days. Many infections are subclinical. Clinical features include: sore throat pharyngeal ulcers, usually resembling herpetic ulcers but affecting posterior mouth alone (soft palate and uvula) (Fig. 38); no gingivitis; cervical lymphadenitis (moderate); fever; malaise, irritability, anorexia, vomiting.

Investigations/
Diagnosis

Clinical diagnosis. Serology (theoretically) is confirmatory. Differentiate from herpetic stomatitis, chickenpox.

Treatment

Symptomatic (see herpes simplex, p. 29).

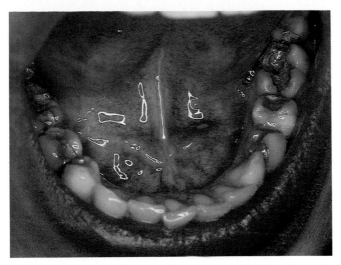

Fig. 37 Hand-foot-and-mouth disease: ulcers indistinguishable from those of herpes simplex.

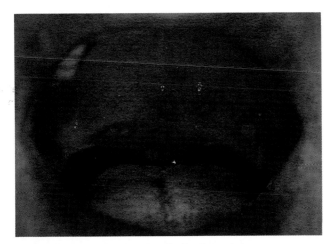

Fig. 38 Herpangina: multiple ulcers of soft palate and pharynx.

Infectious mononucleosis

Common: predominantly a disease of adolescents. Epstein–Barr virus (EBV).

Clinical features

Incubation period probably 15–21 days. Many infections are subclinical. The spectrum of manifestations includes: sore throat, faucial swelling and ulceration with creamy exudate and palatal petechiae; occasional mouth ulcers (Figs 39 & 40); lymph node enlargement—generalized tender lymphadenopathy; fever, malaise, anorexia and lassitude.

*Investigations/
Diagnosis*

Clinical features; blood picture; Paul–Bunnell test for heterophil antibodies. Differentiate from other glandular-like fever syndromes, especially early HIV infection, cytomegalovirus infection, *Toxoplasma gondii* infection and diphtheria.

Treatment

Symptomatic (see herpes simplex, p. 29); metronidazole may improve sore throat.

Measles

*Incidence/
Aetiology*

Common childhood exanthem. Measles virus.

Clinical features

Incubation period 7–14 days. Many infections are subclinical. Features include: Koplik's spots—small white spots on buccal mucosa during prodrome (Fig. 41); rash—maculopapular; conjunctivitis, runny nose, cough; fever, malaise and anorexia.

*Investigations/
Diagnosis*

Clinical features; rising antibody titre confirmatory. Differentiate from thrush, Fordyce spots (not in children).

Treatment

Symptomatic (see herpes simplex, p. 29).

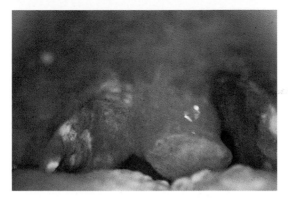

Fig. 39 Infectious mononucleosis: oedema and ulceration of uvula, and tonsillar exudate.

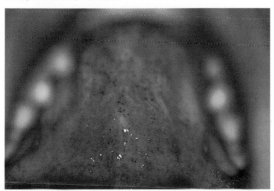

Fig. 40 Infectious mononucleosis: pinpoint haemorrhages (petechiae) of soft palate.

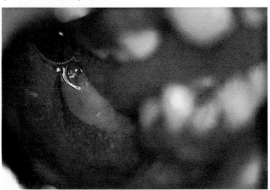

Fig. 41 Measles: Koplik's spots in buccal mucosa.

Acute ulcerative gingivitis (acute necrotizing gingivitis)

Incidence/ Aetiology

Uncommon in developed world. Seen mainly in lower socioeconomic groups, among young male adults. Anaerobic fusiform bacteria and spirochaetes (see also p. 131). Predisposing factors include poor oral hygiene, smoking, (rarely) immune defects and HIV infection.

Clinical features

Ulcers at tips of interdental papillae, occasionally spread along margins (Figs 42 and 147, p. 132); soreness; gingival bleeding; halitosis; rarely fever, malaise, anorexia or cervical lymph node enlargement.

Investigations/ Diagnosis

Clinical diagnosis. Smear may help. Differentiate from leukaemia, herpetic stomatitis.

Treatment

Oral debridement and hygiene instruction. Peroxide or perborate mouthwashes. Metronidazole (penicillin in pregnant females). Periodontal opinion.

Tuberculosis

Incidence/ Aetiology

Uncommon in West. Mainly affects alcoholics, diabetics, patients with immune defects (including HIV infection), and certain racial groups (e.g. Asians). Mycobacteria: usually *M. tuberculosis*, but rarely atypical mycobacteria, e.g. *M. avium-intracellulare*, *M. scrofulaceum*, *M. kansasii*, especially in HIV infection.

Clinical features

Ulceration: usually single chronic ulcer on dorsum of tongue associated with (postprimary) pulmonary infection (Fig. 43).

Investigations/ Diagnosis

Biopsy; sputum culture; chest radiography. Differentiate from other causes of mouth ulcers, especially syphilis and carcinoma (see p. 23).

Treatment

Combination antimicrobial chemotherapy for pulmonary infection. If effective, no local treatment needed.

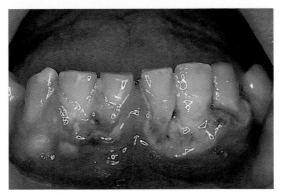

Fig. 42 Acute ulcerative gingivitis: ulceration of interdental papillae and gingival margins.

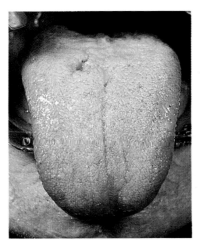

Fig. 43 Tuberculosis: typical pale stellate ulcer on dorsum of tongue.

Syntax

Syphilis

*Incidence/
Aetiology*

Uncommon. *Treponema pallidum*: sexually transmitted. It is predominantly an infection of the sexually active. Other treponematoses, including yaws, bejel and pinta, are rare in the developed world.

Clinical features

Incubation period 9–90 days.

Congenital syphilis
- *Head and neck*: frontal bossing, saddle nose, Hutchinsonian incisors, Moon's or mulberry molars and rhagades (see p. 149).
- *Others*: mental handicap, interstitial keratitis, deafness, sabre tibiae and Clutton's joints.

Acquired syphilis. Stages:
- *Primary syphilis* (see p. 3). Chancre: hard painless papule or nodule that may ulcerate, and heals in 6–8 weeks. It is highly infectious, and usually on genitals or perianally, but rarely on lip or tongue. There is regional lymph node enlargement.
- *Secondary syphilis*. Oral lesions: mucous patches, split papules or snail-track ulcers (Fig. 44). These are highly infectious. Rash (coppery coloured typically on palms and soles), condylomata lata and generalized lymph node enlargement can also be present.
- *Tertiary syphilis*. Oral lesions: glossitis (leukoplakia) and gumma (usually midline in palate or tongue, Fig. 45). These are non-infectious, and may be associated with cardiovascular complications (aortic aneurysm) or neurosyphilis (tabes dorsalis; general paralysis of the insane; Argyll–Robinson pupils).

*Investigations/
Diagnosis*

Direct smear of primary and secondary stage lesions. Serology becomes positive late in primary stage.

Treatment

Penicillin by injection (or erythromycin or tetracycline).

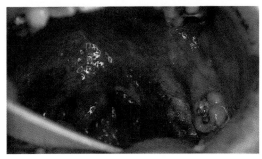

Fig. 44 Syphilis: secondary syphilis showing mucous patches.

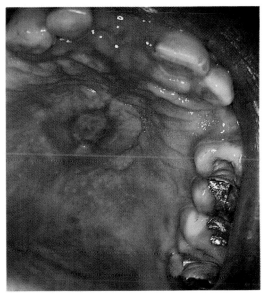

Fig. 45 Gumma (early stage).

Drugs causing mouth ulcers

Incidence/
Aetiology

Ulcers are common in those on cytotoxic drugs.
Other reactions are uncommon or rare. A wide
spectrum of drugs can occasionally cause mouth
ulcers, by various obscure mechanisms. The more
common examples include:
- Cytotoxic agents, particularly methotrexate
- Drugs producing lichen-planus-like (lichenoid)
  lesions, such as antihypertensives, antidiabetics,
  gold salts, non-steroidal anti-inflammatory
  agents, antimalarials and other drugs (Figs 46 &
  47)
- Drugs causing local chemical burns (especially
  aspirin held in the mouth).

Clinical features

- *Drug-induced ulcers*: non-specific.
- *Lichenoid lesions*: resemble lichen planus
  clinically and histologically.
- *Chemical burns*: usually solitary lesions with
  sloughing of mucosa.

Investigations/
Diagnosis

Drug history: test effect of withdrawal.

Treatment

Stop causative drug if possible; symptomatic.

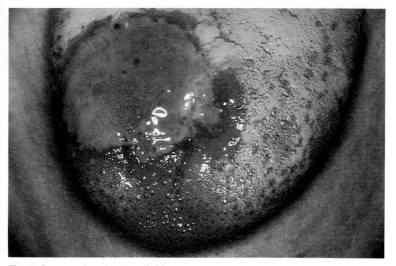

Fig. 46 Drug reaction: due to methyldopa.

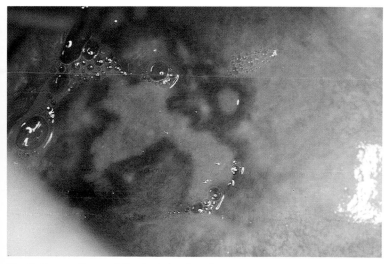

Fig. 47 Drug reaction: penicillamine-induced erosions.

Leukopenia

Incidence/
Aetiology

Uncommon: but lymphopenia due to HIV infection is increasingly common. Viral infections (especially HIV infection), drugs, irradiation, autoimmune, idiopathic.

Clinical features

Predisposition to:
- *infections*—mucosal, systemic or post-operative
- *mouth ulcers*—characteristically persistent ulcers lacking inflammatory halo (Fig. 48).

Investigations/
Diagnosis

Full blood picture; bone marrow biopsy if appropriate. Differentiate from other causes of mouth ulcers (see p. 23), especially leukaemia.

Treatment

Improve oral hygiene; antimicrobials as necessary. $\pm$ Granulocyte colony stimulating factor.

Leukaemia

Incidence/
Aetiology

Uncommon. Idiopathic, irradiation, some chromosomal disorders, chemicals, viruses (see also pp. 7 & 127).

Clinical features

Generalized lymph node enlargement; pallor; hepatosplenomegaly; purpura; oral ulcers (Fig. 49); cervical lymph node enlargement; petechiae and gingival haemorrhage; infections—candidosis or herpetic; others—gingival swelling (acute myeloid leukaemia), labial anaesthesia and facial palsy (rarely) (see also p. 7).

Investigations/
Diagnosis

Full blood picture and bone marrow biopsy. Differentiate from other causes of mouth ulcers (see p. 23) and lymph node enlargement (see p. 143).

Treatment

Chemotherapy and/or bone marrow transplant for leukaemia; supportive care—oral hygiene and topical analgesics aciclovir for herpetic infections; antifungals for candidosis.

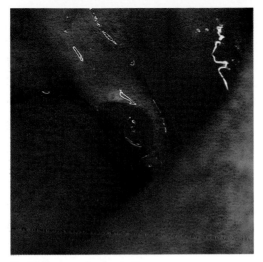

Fig. 48 Neutropenia: ulcer in fauces.

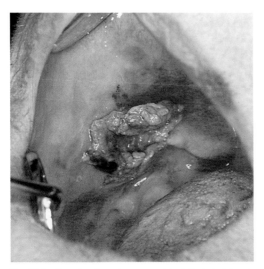

Fig. 49 Leukaemia: ulceration covered by infected clot and exudate.

Malignant tumours

Most malignant oral ulcers are squamous cell carcinomas: the incidence may be rising in some countries. Other primary tumours can be antral (rarely), or of salivary glands, or others, e.g. lymphomas, Kaposi's sarcoma or metastases (see also pp. 5 & 69).

Aetiology

The aetiology of oral carcinoma is unclear. Tobacco and/or alcohol (in some countries) and potentially malignant conditions (dysplastic leukoplakias, candidosis, tertiary syphilis, lichen planus, oral submucous fibrosis and Paterson–Kelly syndrome) may predispose to carcinoma.

Clinical features

Carcinomas present as ulcers, red or white lesions, lumps or fissures, and usually form chronic indurated ulcers typically with raised rolled edge and granulating floor (Figs 50 & 51). Lymphomas (Fig. 52) and Kaposi's sarcoma (Fig. 87, p. 80) are uncommon, but mainly seen in HIV disease.

Investigations/ Diagnosis

Biopsy. Differentiate from other causes of mouth ulcers (see p. 23), especially major aphthae or, rarely, chronic infections, e.g. tuberculosis.

Treatment

Oral carcinoma is treated by one or more of the following: surgery, irradiation and, occasionally, chemotherapy. The prognosis of intraoral carcinoma is poor—about 30% 5-year survival rate. This is because of the high proportion of late stage cases.

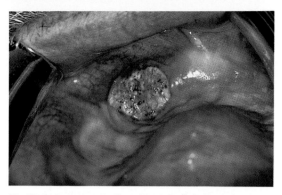

Fig. 50 Oral squamous cell carcinoma: early lesion.

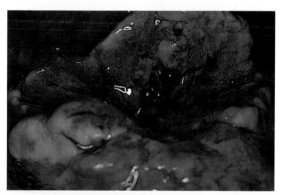

Fig. 51 Oral carcinoma: advanced lesion.

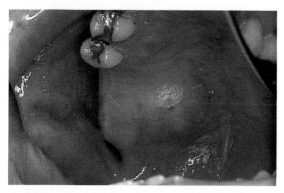

Fig. 52 Lymphoma of palate: ulceration not a feature unless traumatized.

Orofacial granulomatosis

Incidence/ Aetiology

Uncommon. Unknown aetiology; reaction to diet or food additives in some.

Clinical features

Ulcers, typically solitary, persistent and ragged with hyperplastic margins (Fig. 53); there may be other features, particularly facial or labial swelling, tags and/or gingival hyperplasia.

Investigations/ Diagnosis

Biopsy; full blood picture; gastrointestinal studies if necessary. Differentiate from other causes of mouth ulcers (see p. 23), especially malignant lesions or chronic bacterial infections.

Treatment

Antigen exclusion. Topical or intralesional corticosteroids; systemic or possibly topical sulphasalazine.

Ulcerative colitis

Incidence/ Aetiology

Uncommon. Aphthae or other ulcers can be associated with ulcerative colitis by direct cause and effect relationship, or may be secondary to anaemia due to chronic bowel haemorrhage.

Clinical features

General: persistent diarrhoea, frequently painless with passage of blood and mucus in severe cases; iron deficiency anaemia; weight loss.

Oral: mucosal pustules (pyostomatitis vegetans) or irregular chronic ulcers (Fig. 54).

Investigations/ Diagnosis

Biopsy; full blood picture; sigmoidoscopy; barium enema. Differentiate from other causes of mouth ulcers (see p. 23), particularly Crohn's disease.

Treatment

Haematinics for any secondary deficiencies; topical corticosteroids may be helpful; sulphasalazine.

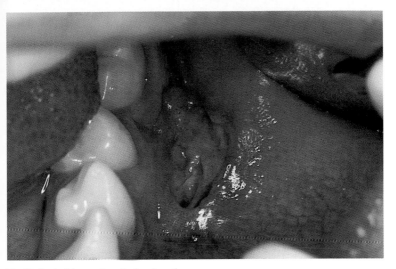

Fig. 53 Orofacial granulomatosis: ulceration.

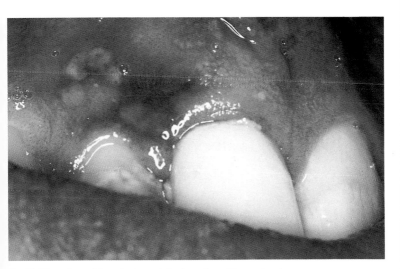

Fig. 54 Ulcerative colitis: minute pustules (pyostomatitis vegetans).

Pemphigus

*Incidence/
Aetiology*

Rare. It is mainly a disease of middle-aged women, especially Mediterranean extraction. Autoimmune: circulating autoantibodies to epithelial intercellular substance. Rarely caused by drugs (penicillamine) or other agents.

Clinical features

Oral lesions are most common in pemphigus vulgaris and often precede skin lesions. Blisters anywhere on the mucosa rupture rapidly to leave ragged ulcers (Figs 55 & 56). Nikolsky's sign is positive. Skin lesions: large flaccid blisters especially where there is trauma. Lesions may affect other mucosae.

*Investigations/
Diagnosis*

- Biopsy to show acantholysis, including immunofluorescence to show IgG and C3 binding to intercellular attachments of epithelial cells.
- Serology (antibodies to intercellular adhesion molecule, desmoglein 3).

Differentiate from other causes of mouth ulcers (see p. 23), especially mucous membrane pemphigoid.

Treatment

Immunosuppression with corticosteroids plus azathioprine or gold.

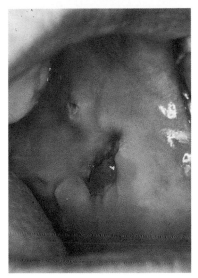

Fig. 55 Pemphigus vulgaris.

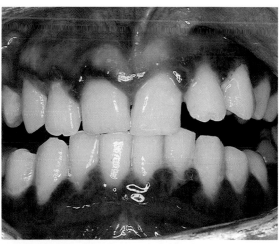

Fig. 56 Pemphigus vulgaris.

Mucous membrane pemphigoid

Incidence/ Aetiology

Not uncommon. Mainly affects middle-aged or elderly females. Has some autoimmune features.

Clinical features

Oral: blisters (sometimes blood-filled) can present anywhere, but especially at sites of trauma. Nikolsky's sign is often positive. Ulcers: may heal with scarring (Figs 57 & 58). 'Desquamative gingivitis' is common (see p. 133).

Others: conjunctival lesions—leading to impaired sight (entropion or symblepharon); laryngeal lesions—may lead to stenosis; skin lesions—blisters rarely (unlike bullous pemphigoid which rarely affects the mouth).

Investigations/ Diagnosis

Biopsy—subepithelial split, including immunostaining (C3 and IgG at basement membrane). Differentiate from other causes of mouth ulcers (see p. 23), especially pemphigus and localized oral purpura.

Treatment

Potent topical corticosteroids or, rarely, systemic corticosteroids or dapsone.

Localized oral purpura

Incidence/ Aetiology

Not uncommon; seen mainly in the elderly. Unclear aetiology, minor or local trauma probably.

Clinical features

Blood blisters in mouth and pharynx, mainly on the soft palate (sometimes termed angina bullosa haemorrhagica) and occasionally on the lateral border of the tongue (Fig. 59). There is rapid onset, with breakdown in a day or two to ulcer. No bleeding tendency.

Investigations/ Diagnosis

Confirm normal haemostasis, biopsy (rarely) to exclude pemphigoid. Differentiate from pemphigoid and other vesiculobullous disorders, trauma, purpura (see also p. 81).

Treatment

Reassure. Topical analgesics.

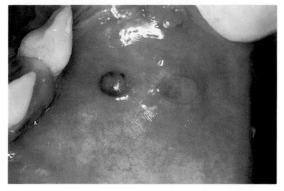

Fig. 57 Mucous membrane pemphigoid (blister).

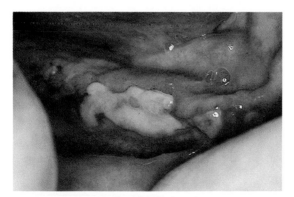

Fig. 58 Mucous membrane pemphigoid: typical erosions

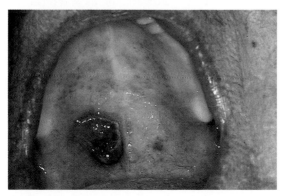

Fig. 59 Localized oral purpura (angina bullosa haemorrhagica): partially ruptured blood blister.

Epidermolysis bullosa

*Incidence/
Aetiology*

Rare. Genetic mostly, including various autosomal dominant (relatively benign) and recessive (more severe) forms. Defect of epithelial basement membrane protein is seen in some subtypes. An acquired form has also been described.

Clinical features

Autosomal dominant forms: skin blisters after trauma, which heal without scars. Oral lesions are rare.

Recessive forms: skin and mouth bullae in neonates (Figs 60 & 61), which heal slowly and scar. Some die; others improve slowly (see also p. 149).

*Investigations/
Diagnosis*

Family history; biopsy to exclude other blistering diseases. Differentiate from other vesiculobullous disorders.

Treatment

Avoid trauma. Phenytoin may benefit some. Corticosteroids are possibly helpful.

Erythema multiforme

Clinical features

Usually attacks for 10–14 days once or twice per year (see also p. 7).

Oral: cracked, bleeding, crusted, swollen lips and ulcers (see Figs 9 & 10, p. 8).

Others: conjunctival and/or genital ulcers; rashes— typically 'target' or 'iris' lesions, or bullae on extremities; fever and malaise.

Mucocutaneous lesions and systemic illness (Stevens–Johnson syndrome): bullous and other rashes, pneumonia, arthritis, nephritis or myocarditis.

*Investigations/
Diagnosis*

Biopsy if needed to exclude other disorders. Differentiate from other oculomucocutaneous syndromes, especially pemphigoid and Behçet's syndrome.

Treatment

See page 7.

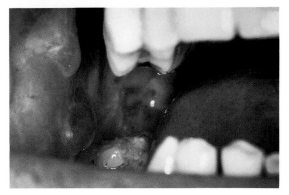

Fig. 60 Epidermolysis bullosa: intact bullae in autosomal dominant form.

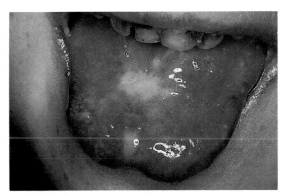

Fig. 61 Epidermolysis bullosa: scarring and secondary depapillation.

Lupus erythematosus

Incidence/ Aetiology

Uncommon. Connective tissue disease (autoimmune) (see also p. 9). Both discoid (DLE) and systemic lupus (SLE) can affect the mouth, and oral lesions can precede other manifestations in a minority of patients.

Clinical features

DLE: characteristic features of intraoral lesions include: central erythema, white spots or papules, radiating white striae at margins and peripheral telangiectasia.

SLE: lesions resemble those in DLE but usually more severe ulceration (Fig. 62). SLE may also be associated with Sjögren syndrome (see p. 139) and, rarely, TMJ arthritis.

Investigations/ Diagnosis

Biopsy; blood picture; Antinuclear factors (crithidial double-stranded DNA) are present in SLE, not DLE.

DLE: differentiate from other causes of mouth ulcers (see p. 23) and especially from SLE, lichen planus and leukoplakia.

SLE: differentiate from other causes of mouth ulcers especially DLE (see p. 23).

Treatment

DLE: topical corticosteroids (rarely systemic).

SLE: systemic steroids, azathioprine, chloroquine or gold.

Lichen planus

This usually causes white lesions and is therefore discussed on page 57. However, it can present with erosions (Fig. 63).

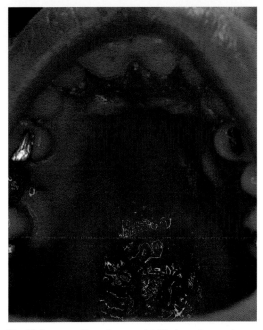

Fig. 62 Lupus erythematosus: palatal lesions at an early stage of SLE.

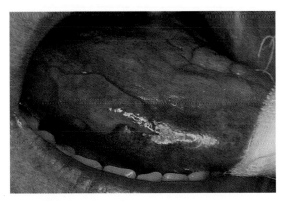

Fig. 63 Lichen planus: erosion with faint peripheral striae.

Lichen planus

Incidence/
Aetiology

Common; mainly middle-aged or elderly females (see also p. 9). Usually no aetiological factor is identifiable. A minority are due to drugs (lichenoid lesions, see p. 41), graft-versus-host disease, HIV infection, liver disorders (possibly) and reactions to amalgam or gold (possibly).

Clinical features

Sometimes asymptomatic. White striate lesions are common (Figs 64 & 65); erosions are less common. Lesions tend to be bilateral.

Reticular lesions are most often found on buccal mucosa, sometimes on the tongue. Papular lesions affect similar sites. Plaque-like lesions usually affect posterior buccal mucosa. Red lesions of atrophic LP may simulate erythroplasia (see p. 79). LP can cause 'desquamative gingivitis' (see p. 133). Oral lesions are occasionally hyperpigmented. Rash: pruritic, polygonal, purplish papules predominantly on flexor surfaces of wrists, and shins, rarely on the face. Trauma may induce lesions (Koebner phenomenon). Genital lesions, alopecia or nail deformities are seen occasionally.

Erosions are irregular, persistent and painful, with yellowish slough, and are often associated with white lesions (see Fig. 63, p. 56). It may have a small malignant potential (1% ± after 10 years).

Investigations/
Diagnosis

Drug history; biopsy. Differentiate from other white lesions (see p. 69) and ulcers (see p. 23), especially DLE and keratoses.

Treatment

- *Asymptomatic*: no treatment.
- *Symptomatic*: corticosteroids topically and, rarely, intralesionally or systemically. Other drugs such as retinoids, griseofulvin or cyclosporin have not proved reliably superior, or may have adverse effects.

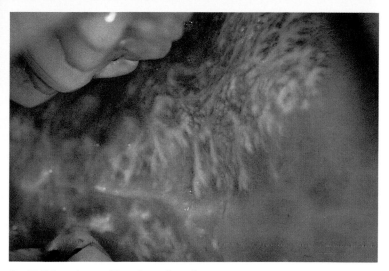

Fig. 64 Lichen planus: white striae and papules.

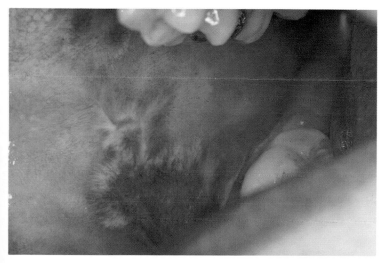

Fig. 65 Lichen planus: atrophic area with peripheral striae.

Candidosis

Incidence/
Aetiology

Thrush

Disturbed oral microflora by antibiotics, corticosteroids or xerostomia; immune defects, especially in HIV infection, immunosuppressive treatment, leukaemias and lymphomas, and diabetes. Rare in healthy patients except neonates.

Clinical features

White or creamy plaques that can be wiped off to leave a red base (Fig. 66).

Investigations/
Diagnosis

Gram stain smear (hyphae); blood picture. Differentiate from Koplik's or Fordyce's spots and lichen planus.

Treatment

Treat predisposing cause. Antifungals: nystatin oral suspension *or* pastilles *or* amphotericin lozenges *or* miconazole gel or tablets, *or* fluconazole tablets.

Incidence/
Aetiology

Chronic mucocutaneous candidosis

Rare. Immune defects sometimes; occasionally genetic; HIV infection.

Clinical features

Oral: persistent widespread leukoplakia (Fig. 67).

Cutaneous: nail and skin candidosis.

Others: rarely familial multiple endocrinopathies, iron deficiency or thymoma.

Investigations/
Diagnosis

Family history; biopsy; blood picture; auto-antibody and endocrine studies. Differentiate from other white lesions (see p. 69).

Treatment

Antifungals (as above) including systemic fluconazole or itraconazole.

Incidence/
Aetiology

Candidal leukoplakia (limited type)

The condition is uncommon, but considerably more common than chronic mucocutaneous candidosis. Smoking predisposes.

Clinical features

Leukoplakia is typically found at commissures, often speckled. There may be a higher malignant potential than many leukoplakias (see also Fig. 73, p. 66).

Investigations/
Diagnosis

Biopsy. Differentiate from other oral white lesions (see p. 69).

Treatment

Antifungals; stop smoking; biopsy, and remove (excision, laser or cryosurgery) *or* observe.

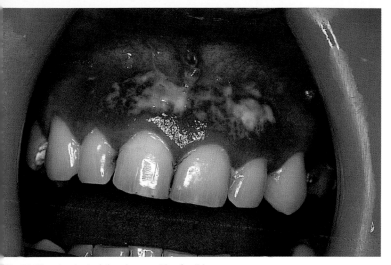

Fig. 66 Thrush: gingival thrush caused by *C. albicans*.

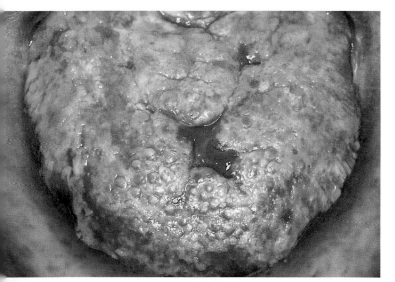

Fig. 67 Chronic mucocutaneous candidosis: widespread adherent plaque.

Chemical burns

Incidence/
Aetiology
Common. Various chemicals or drugs, notably aspirin put in sulcus to try to relieve toothache.

Clinical features
White lesion with sloughing mucosa localized usually to buccal sulcus and adjacent buccal mucosa, often beside carious tooth (Fig. 68).

Investigations/
Diagnosis
History. Differentiate from other white lesions (see p. 69).

Treatment
Treat toothache as appropriate. Stop the habit: lesion is self-healing.

Cheek biting

Incidence/
Aetiology
Common: most prevalent in anxious females, especially those with other psychologically related disorders, e.g. temporomandibular pain-dysfunction syndrome. Rarely (self-mutilation) seen in psychiatric disorders, mental handicap or some rare syndromes. See also frictional keratosis, page 65.

Clinical features
Abrasion of superficial epithelium leaves whitish fragments on reddish background (Fig. 69). Lesions are invariably restricted to lower labial mucosa and/or buccal mucosa near occlusal line.

Diagnosis
Clinical features. Differentiate from other causes of white lesions (see p. 69), particularly white sponge naevus.

Treatment
Stop the habit if possible.

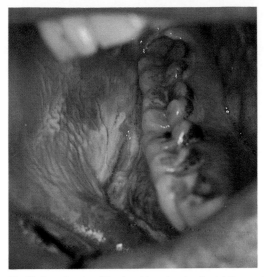

Fig. 68 Burn from aspirin placed in sulcus in attempt to relieve pain from carious tooth.

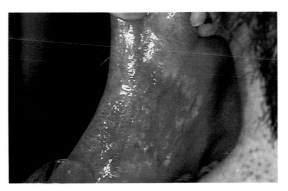

Fig. 69 Cheek biting.

Keratoses

Leukoplakia is the term used for hyperkeratotic white mucosal lesions of unknown cause. There are no specific histopathological connotations.

Fairly common. Keratoses are seen mainly in middle-aged/elderly adults, but hairy leukoplakia is seen mainly in young adult males.

Idiopathic: most cases (Fig. 70).

Friction (Fig. 71).

Tobacco: pipe smoking can cause 'nicotinic stomatitis' of palate especially; smokeless tobacco or betel-chewing can cause keratosis, usually of buccal sulcus (see Fig. 72, p. 66).

Microorganisms
- *Candida albicans.* Candidal leukoplakias frequently appear speckled, often affect commissures and may have fairly high malignant potential (see Fig. 73, p. 66).
- *Syphilis.* Syphilitic leukoplakias especially affect the dorsum of tongue and have high malignant potential (see Fig. 74, p. 68).
- *'Hairy' leukoplakia* is virtually pathognomonic of HIV infection. Epstein–Barr virus may be detected. It is not premalignant (see Fig. 75, p. 68).
- *Focal epithelial hyperplasia* (Heck's disease) is rare. Predominantly affects Eskimos and American Indians and is caused by human papillomavirus. ➡

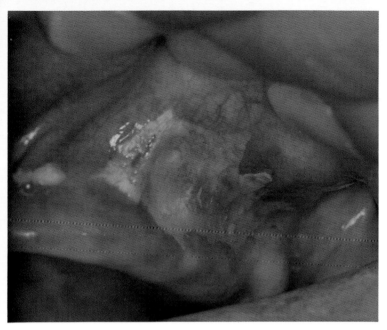

Fig. 70 Homogeneous leukoplakia.

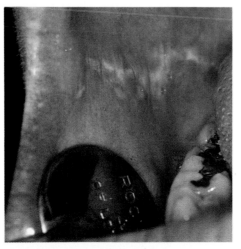

Fig. 71 Occlusal line caused by friction.

Most keratoses are benign, but overall 1–3% are premalignant. Keratoses in particular sites or of particular appearance tend to have higher premalignant potential, but epithelial dysplasia, microscopically, is a more reliable guide.

Sites: most frequently in the buccal mucosa.

Appearance: most are smooth plaques (homogeneous leukoplakias, Fig. 70, p. 64); some warty (verrucous leukoplakia); some mixed white and red lesions (speckled leukoplakias). In general, homogeneous leukoplakias are benign, malignant potential is higher in verrucous leukoplakias, and is highest in speckled leukoplakias. Some studies show malignant transformation in over 20% of speckled leukoplakias.

Frictional keratosis.   Usually seen at sites of trauma from teeth, also along buccal occlusal line (Fig. 71, p. 64) and occasionally beside an outstanding tooth, or on edentulous ridge. It is homogeneous and clears up when irritation is removed.

Smoker's keratosis ('stomatitis nicotina').   Pipe smoking is the usual cause. The palate, particularly the soft palate, is affected. Red orifices of swollen minor salivary glands of palate within widespread white lesion give striking appearance of red spots on white background (Fig. 72). This lesion is benign in itself, but carcinoma may develop nearby.

Other tobacco-related habits.   Tobacco-chewing, snuff-dipping or chewing of betel quids may lead to keratoses which can be premalignant. Snuff-dipping is associated predominantly with verrucous keratoses which can progress to verrucous carcinoma (p. 97). Smokeless tobacco is likely to have the same effect. Tobacco-related keratoses typically resolve on stopping the habit. ➥

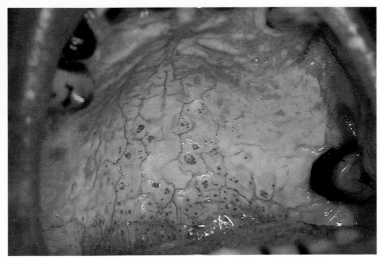

Fig. 72 Smoker's keratosis: showing inflamed orifices of minor palatal glands.

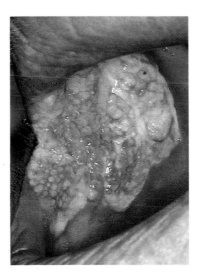

Fig. 73 Speckled leukoplakia (chronic candidosis in this case).

Clinical types (cont.)	*Candidal leukoplakia.* *C. albicans* can cause or colonize other keratoses, particularly in smokers, and is especially likely to form speckled leukoplakias at commissures (see Fig. 78, p. 72). It may be dysplastic and have higher malignant potential than some other keratoses. Candidal leukoplakias may respond to antifungals and stopping smoking. *Syphilitic leukoplakias.* Leukoplakia, especially of the dorsum of tongue, is a feature of tertiary syphilis but rare (Fig. 74). Malignant potential is high. *Hairy leukoplakia.* Usually has a corrugated surface and affects margins of the tongue almost exclusively (Fig. 75). It is seen in the immunocompromised and is a complication of HIV infection and a predictor of those who will progress to full-blown AIDS. The condition is benign, and self-limiting or may respond to aciclovir. *Leukoplakia in chronic renal failure.* Symmetrical soft keratosis may complicate chronic renal failure, but resolves after treatment by renal transplantation or dialysis. *Sublingual keratosis.* Keratoses in the floor of the mouth/ventrum of tongue were formerly thought to be naevi (congenital) but, although of unknown aetiology, are reported to have malignant potential higher than other leukoplakias. A few studies suggest that >20% undergo malignant transformation. Often homogeneous, there may be speckled areas. The surface has an 'ebbing tide' appearance (see Fig. 76, p. 70). Opinions vary as to whether the lesion should be left undisturbed or removed surgically or by laser or cryoprobe.
Investigations/ Diagnosis	Most white lesions need to be biopsied for possible dysplasia or early malignant change.

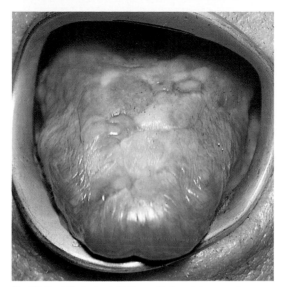

Fig. 74 Syphilis: leukoplakia/depapillation of dorsum of tongue in tertiary syphilis.

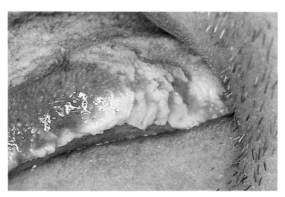

Fig. 75 AIDS. Hairy leukoplakia showing the more common corrugated appearance.

Differentiate from other oral white lesions:

Developmental
- White sponge naevus.
- Other rare syndromes.

Acquired
- Transient—burns, cheek-biting. Thrush.
- Persistent—keratosis (frictional, idiopathic, smoker's, candidal, syphilitic); thrush in HIV.
- Lichen planus.
- Lupus erythematosus.
- Carcinoma.

Treatment

See above but in general:
- treat any predisposing factors
- surgically remove small discrete lesions <2 cm diameter
- observe regularly larger lesions.

Carcinoma

Keratinizing carcinomas may appear as oral white lesions (Fig. 77) *ab initio* or may occasionally arise in other oral white lesions, notably in some keratoses, dyskeratosis congenita, oral submucous fibrosis, or rarely in lichen planus (see also pp. 5 & 45).

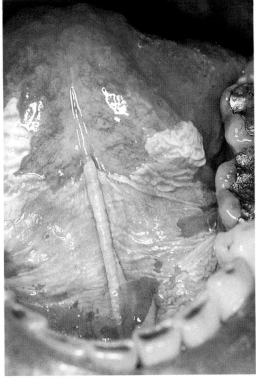

Fig. 76 Sublingual keratosis with typical wrinkled surface.

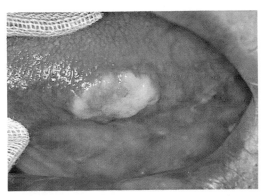

Fig. 77 Squamous cell carcinoma (early stage producing small white patch).

White sponge naevus

*Incidence/
Aetiology*

Rare: often recognized later in life. Genetic: autosomal dominant, but family history may be negative.

Clinical features

Oral lesions predominate: asymptomatic, diffuse, bilateral white lesions with shaggy or spongy, wrinkled surface (Fig. 78). They mainly present on the buccal mucosa, but sometimes on the tongue, floor of mouth, or elsewhere, and may involve the pharynx, oesophagus, nose, genitals and anus.

*Investigations/
Diagnosis*

Clinical features; biopsy is confirmatory. Differentiate from other white lesions (see p. 69), especially cheek biting.

Treatment

Reassurance.

Oral submucous fibrosis (OSMF)

*Incidence/
Aetiology*

Virtually only a disease of adults from Indian sub-continent, related to the use of areca nuts.

Clinical features

Tight vertical bands in buccal mucosa (Fig. 79) that may progress to severely restrict oral opening. It can also affect the palate or tongue. Often anaemia is present. Malignant potential—carcinoma possibly in up to 25%.

*Investigations/
Diagnosis*

Clinical features; biopsy; haematology. Differentiate from scleroderma (see p. 73).

Treatment

Stop use of areca nut.

Asymptomatic: observe only.

Symptomatic with restricted opening: exercises, intralesional corticosteroids, surgery. Possibly penicillamine.

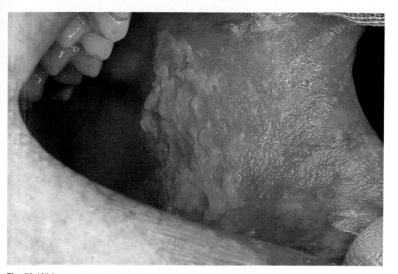

Fig. 78 White sponge naevus.

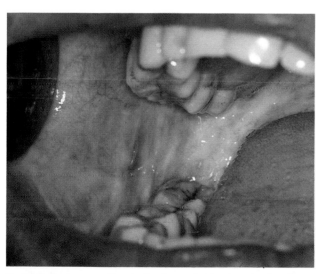

Fig. 79 Oral submucous fibrosis showing vertical bands and pallor of mucosa.

Hereditary haemorrhagic telangiectasia (HHT; Osler–Rendu–Weber syndrome)

Incidence/ Aetiology

Rare autosomal dominant condition, but family history may be negative.

Clinical features

Telangiectases are present orally and periorally (Fig. 80) but also in nose, gastrointestinal tract and occasionally on palms. Telangiectases may bleed, resulting in iron deficiency anaemia.

Investigations/ Diagnosis

Clinical features; blood picture. Differentiate from other causes of telangiectasia: scleroderma, chronic liver disease and post-irradiation.

Treatment

Cryosurgery or laser if bleeding is troublesome; treat anaemia.

Scleroderma (systemic sclerosis)

Incidence/ Aetiology

Uncommon: mainly middle-aged females. Probably autoimmune.

Clinical features

Oral: opening restricted with microstoma and pale fibrotic 'chicken' tongue; widened periodontal space on radiography in a few, but teeth not mobile.

Occasionally: telangiectasia (Fig. 81); secondary Sjögren syndrome; bone lesions.

Other features: skin—tight and waxy; Raynaud syndrome; dysphagia.

Rare variant: CRST syndrome (calcinosis, Raynaud syndrome, sclerodactyly, telangiectasia).

Investigations/ Diagnosis

Clinical features; histopathology; auto-antibodies (ANF and Scl 70 especially). Oral lesions: differentiate from OSMF (see p. 71), telangiectasia (e.g. HHT, see above) and secondary Sjögren syndrome (see pp. 119 & 139).

Treatment

Penicillamine.

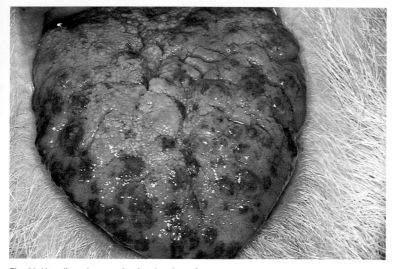

Fig. 80 Hereditary haemorrhagic telangiectasia.

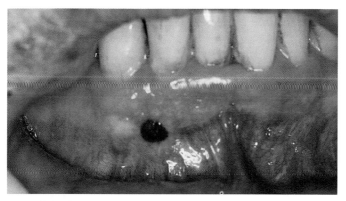

Fig. 81 Scleroderma: single oral telangiectasis.

Haemangioma

*Incidence/
Aetiology*
Common on tongue, vermilion border of lip, or buccal mucosa. Hamartoma or benign tumour.

Clinical features
Red or blue, painless, soft and sometimes fluctuant lesions that usually blanch on pressure (Figs 82, 83 & 122, p. 112). Most appear in infancy.

*Investigations/
Diagnosis*
Aspiration; biopsy (excision if feasible) for confirmation, rarely necessary. Differentiate from telangiectasia, purpura, Kaposi's sarcoma and epithelioid angiomatosis. Rarely: haemangioendotheliomas, Maffucci syndrome (multiple haemangiomas and enchondromas) and Fabry's disease (a lipidosis).

Treatment
Observation (some 50% regress spontaneously), cryosurgery, argon laser, sclerosant or (rarely) arterial embolization—only if bleeding is troublesome.

Sturge–Weber syndrome

*Incidence/
Aetiology*
Rare. Congenital (see also p. 21).

Clinical features
Haemangioma within trigeminal sensory area, extending into leptomeninges; epilepsy; hemiplegia (sometimes); mentally challenged (common).

*Investigations/
Diagnosis*
Clinical features; skull radiograph (intracerebral calcification). Differentiate from isolated haemangioma and other rare syndromes.

Treatment
Anticonvulsants for epilepsy.

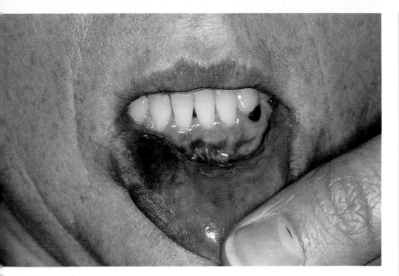

Fig. 82 Haemangioma.

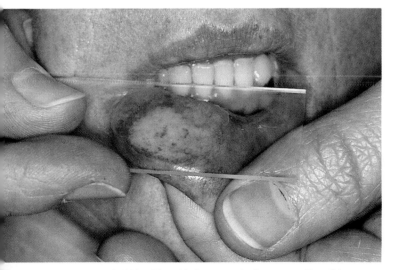

Fig. 83 Haemangioma: typical blanching of lesion as result of pressure with a slide.

Radiation-induced lesions

Aetiology

Invariable if teletherapy (external beam treatment) involves oral mucosa and salivary glands.

Clinical features

Mucositis: diffuse erythema and ulceration (Fig. 84).

Xerostomia: leading to dysphagia, disturbed taste, candidosis, sialadenitis, radiation caries.
Liability to osteoradionecrosis.

Others: Trismus; telangiectasia (late); jaw hypoplasia, hypoplasia and retarded eruption of developing teeth in children.

Diagnosis

Diagnosis clear from history; avoid biopsy.

Treatment

Symptomatic; control infections. Treatment with antimicrobials active against Gram negative bacilli may prevent mucositis.

Denture-induced stomatitis

*Incidence/
Aetiology*

Common: mainly elderly patients. Usually *C. albicans*. Constant denture-wearing predisposes, but other factors may include poor denture hygiene, high carbohydrate diet and HIV infection.

Clinical features

Diffuse erythema of denture-bearing area only (Fig. 85), with occasional petechiae or thrush. Almost always asymptomatic. The only known complications are angular stomatitis (see p. 11) and aggravation of palatal papillary hyperplasia.

*Investigations/
Diagnosis*

Diagnosis is clinical. Smear for hyphae. Differentiate from erythroplasia or trauma.

Treatment

Leave dentures out at night in antifungal (e.g. hypochlorite, chlorhexidine); antifungals; attention to dentures.

Erythematous candidosis

Candidosis may cause sore red mouth especially in patients with xerostomia or on broad spectrum antimicrobials. Erythematous candidosis, especially on the palate or tongue, may also be a feature of HIV disease.

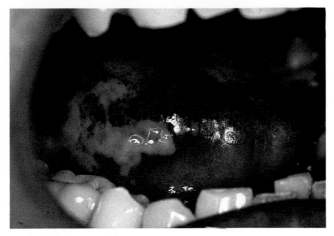

Fig. 84 Radiation mucositis.

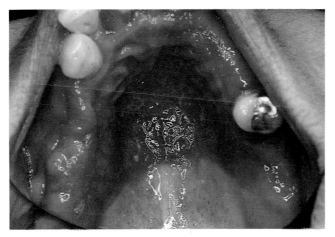

Fig. 85 Denture-induced stomatitis.

Erythroplasia (erythroplakia)

Incidence/ Aetiology

Uncommon: mainly seen in elderly males. It is much less common than leukoplakia, but far more likely to be dysplastic or malignant. Unknown aetiology.

Clinical features

Red velvety patch of variable configuration, commonly on soft palate or floor of mouth. Usually level with or depressed below surrounding mucosa (Fig. 86).

Investigations/ Diagnosis

Biopsy for epithelial dysplasia and carcinoma—present in over 90%. Differentiate from inflammatory and atrophic lesions, e.g. in deficiency anaemias, geographic tongue, lichen planus.

Treatment

Excise, but the prognosis is often poor.

Kaposi's sarcoma

Incidence/ Aetiology

Seen mainly as feature of HIV infection and is a malignant neoplasm of endothelial cells. It is associated with human herpesvirus-8 (HHV-8).

Clinical features

Early lesions are red, purple or brown macules. Later these become nodular, extend, disseminate and may ulcerate. Kaposi's sarcoma typically involves the palate or maxillary gingivae, but can affect any other oral site (Fig. 87).

Investigations/ Diagnosis

Biopsy is confirmatory. Differentiate from other pigmented lesions (see p. 81), especially epithelioid angiomatosis, haemangiomas and purpura.

Treatment

Treatment of underlying predisposing condition if possible; radiotherapy; vinca alkaloids.

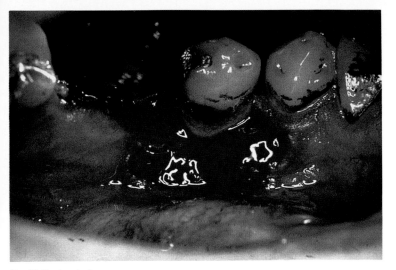

Fig. 86 Erythroplasia.

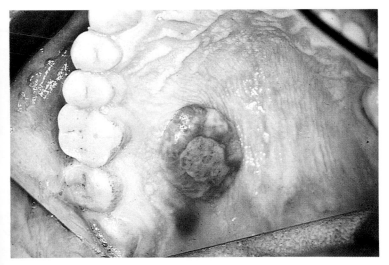

Fig. 87 Kaposi's sarcoma (macule and ulcerated nodule).

Purpura

*Incidence/
Aetiology*

A few traumatic petechiae may be seen at the occlusal line in otherwise healthy persons. Otherwise, oral purpura is uncommon. Platelet deficiency—idiopathic (autoimmune), sometimes in HIV/AIDS; platelet defect; vascular defect rarely; localized oral purpura ('angina bullosa haemorrhagica', see p. 51). Palatal petechiae are a feature of infectious mononucleosis but may be seen in HIV disease or rubella, or where there is vomiting in bulimia.

Clinical features

Red or brown pinpoint lesions (petechiae) or ecchymoses mainly at sites of trauma (Fig. 88). Lesions do not blanch on pressure (cf. haemangioma).

*Investigations/
Diagnosis*

Blood picture (including blood count) and haemostatic function. Differentiate from haemangiomas, telangiectasia and Kaposi's sarcoma. Thrombocytopenia is also seen in HIV infection.

Treatment

Treat the underlying cause.

Racial pigmentation

*Incidence/
Aetiology*

Racial pigmentation is common not only in coloured patients but also in some whites, especially those from Mediterranean littoral.

Clinical features

Brown (rarely black) pigmentation, especially of the gingiva (Fig. 89) or tongue.

*Investigations/
Diagnosis*

Nil unless to exclude Addison's disease (see p. 83). Differentiate from other causes of pigmentation (especially Addison's disease), namely:
- *Localized*: amalgam tattoo, ephelis, naevi, Peutz–Jeghers syndrome, melanoma and Kaposi's sarcoma
- *Generalized*: racial, Addison's disease, drugs and other rare causes including HIV/AIDS.

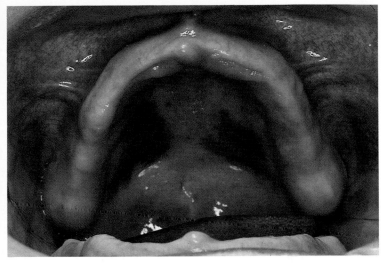

Fig. 88 Purpura of palate due to thrombocytopenia but triggered by pressure of denture.

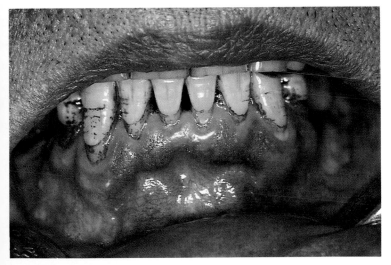

Fig. 89 Racial pigmentation.

Peutz–Jeghers syndrome

See Figure 90 and page 19.

Addison's disease (hypoadrenocorticism)

Incidence/ Aetiology

Rare; mainly a disease of young or middle-aged females, except in AIDS. Adrenocortical destruction causes include autoimmune hypoadrenalism and, rarely, tuberculosis, histoplasmosis (sometimes in AIDS) and carcinomatosis.

Nelson syndrome is similar but iatrogenic and results from adrenalectomy in the management of breast cancer.

Clinical features

Hyperpigmentation, especially in sites usually pigmented or traumatized.

Oral: brown pigmentation of gingiva, occlusal line and elsewhere (Fig. 91).

Cutaneous: hyperpigmentation of areolae and genitals, in flexures, and at sites of trauma.

Rarely: associated with other autoimmune glandular disease; or candidosis-endocrinopathy syndrome.

Investigations/ Diagnosis

Blood pressure; plasma electrolyte and low cortisol levels and response to ACTH (Synacthen test). Differentiate from other causes of pigmentation (see p. 81) especially racial and drugs.

Treatment

Idiopathic (autoimmune) Addison's disease: replacement therapy (fludrocortisone and corticosteroids).
Others: treat cause, give replacement therapy.

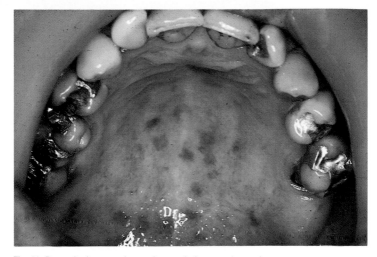

Fig. 90 Peutz–Jeghers syndrome: intraoral pigmented macules.

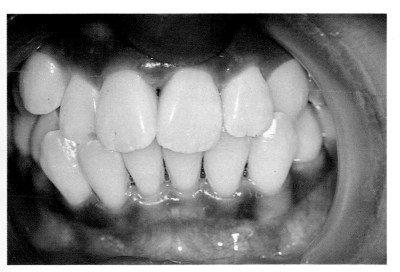

Fig. 91 Addison's hypoadrenocorticism: intraoral pigmentation (clinically indistinguishable from racial type).

Drug-induced hyperpigmentation

Incidence/ Aetiology
Rare. A variety of drugs cause pigmentation rarely, often by unknown mechanisms. Adrenocorticotropic hormone (ACTH) can cause pigmentation by virtue of MSH-like activity. (ACTH-producing neoplasms act similarly.) In the past, heavy metals (e.g. lead) caused pigmented lines because of sulphide deposits in gingival pockets (Fig. 92). Drugs currently implicated include anti-malarials, busulphan, cisplatin, phenothiazines, ACTH, zidovudine and oral contraceptives.

Clinical features
Variable colour, patchy or localized according to cause.

Investigations/ Diagnosis
History of exposure to drug. Differentiate from other causes of pigmentation (see p. 81).

Treatment
Stop the causative drug if possible.

Amalgam tattoo

Incidence/ Aetiology
Common in adults mainly. Amalgam particles or dust can become incorporated in healing wounds after tooth extraction or apicectomy or beneath mucosa.

Clinical features
Black or bluish-black (usually) solitary small pigmented area beneath normal mucosa (Fig. 93); usually related to lower ridge or buccal vestibule. It is asymptomatic and may rarely be radiopaque.

Investigations/ Diagnosis
Excise to exclude melanoma by microscopy. Differentiate from other causes of pigmentation (see p. 81), especially naevi and melanoma.

Treatment
Excision biopsy necessary to distinguish from naevus or melanoma.

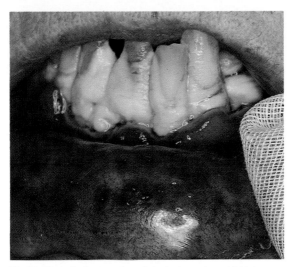

Fig. 92 Bismuth pigmentation of gingival margin and labial glands.

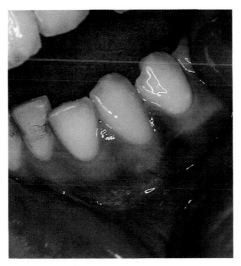

Fig. 93 Amalgam tattoo.

Pigmented naevi

Incidence/
Aetiology

Common. Congenital (see also page 19).

Clinical features

Brownish or bluish macules, usually <1 cm across (Fig. 94). Asymptomatic.

Investigations/
Diagnosis

Biopsy. Differentiate from other causes of pigmentation (see p. 81), especially amalgam tattoo or melanoma.

Treatment

Excision biopsy to exclude malignant melanoma.

Malignant melanoma

Incidence/
Aetiology

Unknown but rare compared with skin. Men are more frequently affected, most often between 40–70 years. Malignant tumour of melanocytes.

Clinical features

Heavily pigmented (Fig. 95) (occasionally non-pigmented) macule or later, nodule and ulceration. It may spread across several cm. The palate is most frequently affected, with spread to regional lymph nodes and then the bloodstream.

Investigations/
Diagnosis

Wide excision biopsy, assessment of invasion depth. Differentiate from naevi and other pigmented lesions (see p. 81).

Treatment

Wide excision, but the prognosis is poor unless treatment is exceptionally early. Hence the need to biopsy all small pigmented lesions.

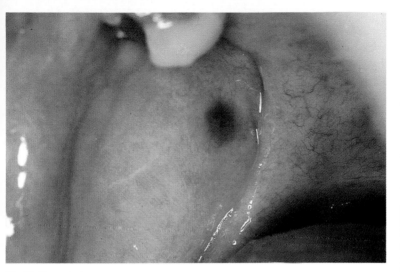

Fig. 94 Pigmented naevus.

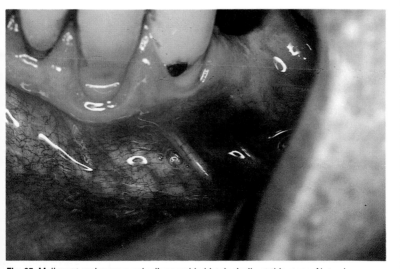

Fig. 95 Malignant melanoma: only diagnosable histologically at this stage. Note also cervical abrasion.

Denture-induced hyperplasia (denture granuloma)

Incidence/ Aetiology

Common: mainly in middle-aged or elderly patients. Pressure from denture flange causes chronic irritation and hyperplastic response. It is usually related to lower complete denture, especially anteriorly (see Fig. 26, p. 24).

Clinical features

Usually seen in the buccal sulcus, occasionally over genial tubercles. A painless lump with smooth pink surface lies parallel with alveolar ridge and may be grooved by denture margins (Figs 96 & 97).

Investigations/ Diagnosis

Excision biopsy. Usually the diagnosis is clearcut if the lesion is in relation to denture flange. If ulcerated, it may mimic carcinoma (rarely).

Treatment

Excise to confirm diagnosis; relieve denture flange to prevent recurrence.

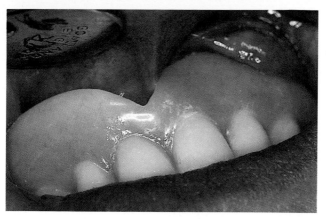

Fig. 96 Denture-induced hyperplasia showing relation to denture flange.

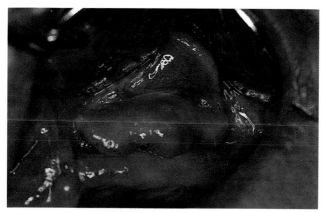

Fig. 97 Denture-induced hyperplasia (same patient) showing fissured conformation.

Fibrous nodules ('fibroepithelial polyp')

Common. Chronic irritation causing fibrous hyperplasia.

Pedunculated or broadly sessile, sometimes ulcerated, hard or soft, mainly on buccal mucosa or elsewhere (Figs 98 & 99). It is termed 'fibrous epulis' if on gingival margin.

Excision biopsy. Differentiate from any other soft tissue tumour.

Excise for histological confirmation.

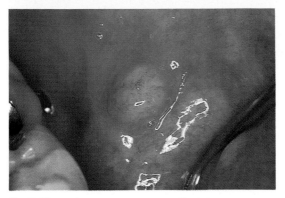

Fig. 98 Fibrous lump: more common sessile variant.

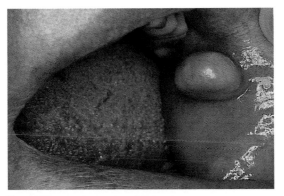

Fig. 99 Fibrous polyp: pedunculated variant.

Lipoma

Incidence/ Aetiology

Rare benign tumour of adipose tissue.

Clinical features

Slow-growing, yellowish, soft, semi-fluctuant, painless mass usually on buccal mucosa (Fig. 100).

Investigations/ Diagnosis

Biopsy. Differentiate from other swellings.

Treatment

Excise.

Lymphangioma

Incidence/ Aetiology

Rare hamartoma or benign neoplasm of lymphatic channels.

Clinical features

Colourless, sometimes finely nodular soft mass. Bleeding into lymphatic spaces causes sudden purplish discolouration. If in tongue and extensive, it is a rare cause of macroglossia (Fig. 101). If in lip, it is a rare cause of macrocheilia.

Investigations/ Diagnosis

Excision biopsy. Differentiate from haemangiomas mainly.

Treatment

Excise for microscopy.

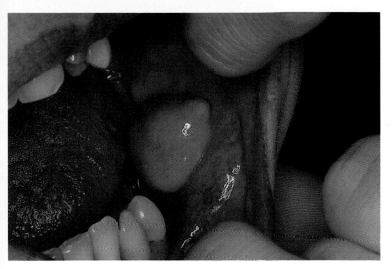

Fig. 100 Lipoma.

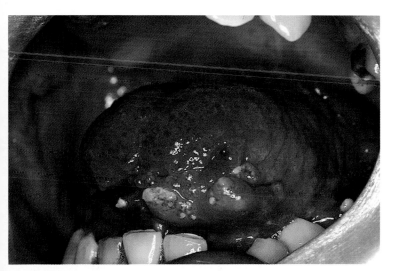

Fig. 101 Lymphangioma causing macroglossia.

Human papillomavirus (HPV) infections

HPV most commonly produce papillomas, but are also implicated in various warts including venereal warts (condyloma acuminatum), and rare disorders, e.g. focal epithelial hyperplasia (Heck's disease), possibly in carcinomas.

Warts

Incidence/ Aetiology

Uncommon. A higher prevalence is seen in patients with sexually transmitted diseases or who are immunocompromised as in HIV/AIDS. Usually transmitted from skin lesions (verruca vulgaris) and occasionally from genital lesions (condyloma acuminata).

Clinical features

Verrucae are found predominantly on the lips (Fig. 102). Condyloma acuminata are found on the tongue or palate. Either can be warty papules or more smooth-surfaced.

Investigations/ Diagnosis

Biopsy. Differentiate from papillomas and other tumours.

Treatment

Excision and microscopy; podophyllin; laser; cryosurgery; intralesional interferon.

Papillomas

Incidence

Most common benign soft tissue neoplasm; usually found in 20–50 year age group.

Clinical features

Most commonly papillated asymptomatic, pedunculated lesion, either pink or white if hyperkeratinized, on palate, tongue or other sites (Fig. 103). They are found also in some rare syndromes.

Investigations/ Diagnosis

Biopsy. Differentiate from warts and other epithelial neoplasms.

Treatment

As for warts (above).

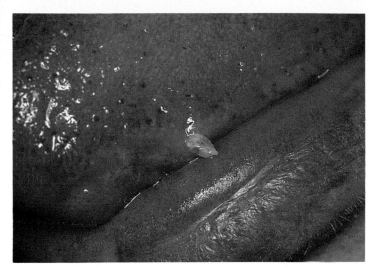

Fig. 102 Wart.

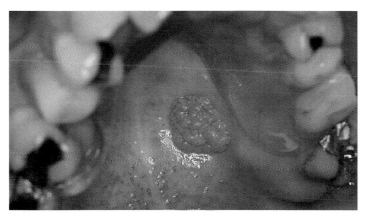

Fig. 103 Papilloma.

Verrucous carcinoma

Carcinoma (p. 45) and other malignant neoplasms may form lumps in mouth. This is especially true in verrucous carcinoma (Fig. 104).

Antral carcinoma

Incidence/ Aetiology

Rare: male predominance, usually seen in elderly. Identified predisposing factor appears to be occupational exposure to wood dust. It is usually a squamous carcinoma.

Clinical features

Initially asymptomatic until carcinoma invades nerves, orbit or other structures to cause paraesthesia, anaesthesia, swelling of cheek or eye area, nasal obstruction or pain. Symptoms depend on main direction of spread.

Oral invasion: pain and swelling of palate, alveolus or sulcus (Fig. 105). Teeth may loosen.

Ocular invasion: ipsilateral epiphora, diplopia or proptosis.

Nasal invasion: nasal obstruction or a blood-stained discharge.

Investigations/ Diagnosis

Biopsy and radiographs. Sinus radiography shows opaque antrum and later destruction of antral wall or floor. Differentiate from sinusitis, polyps and salivary gland neoplasms.

Treatment

Surgery (sometimes with radiotherapy). Prognosis 10–30% 5-year survival; better in those with no lymph node involvement.

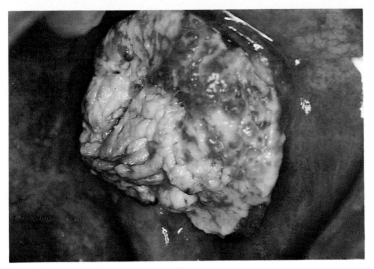

Fig. 104 Verrucous carcinoma with transition to invasive carcinoma.

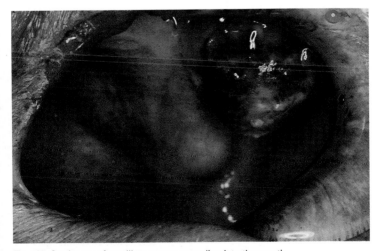

Fig. 105 Carcinoma of maxillary antrum extending into the mouth.

Intraoral salivary gland neoplasms

Incidence/ Aetiology

Rare. Unknown aetiology. Intraoral salivary gland neoplasms are less common than in major glands, but a higher proportion are malignant (see also pp. 45 & 141). Pleomorphic adenoma is the most common intraoral salivary neoplasm, but adenoid cystic carcinoma and mucoepidermoid carcinoma are more common in the mouth than in major glands. Peak prevalence (all types) is seen in older persons, especially females. Intraorally, the palate is the site of predilection. Salivary gland tumours in the tongue are usually malignant—especially adenoid cystic carcinoma. Salivary gland tumours in the lips are usually in the upper lip and typically benign (pleomorphic or monomorphic adenoma). Most tumours of the sublingual gland are malignant.

Clinical features

Benign neoplasms form painless swellings. Pleomorphic adenoma are typically rubbery and often lobulated (Fig. 106).

Malignant tumours in later stages are often painful and ulcerate (Fig. 107); they metastasise to upper cervical lymph nodes. Not initially distinguishable clinically from benign tumours.

Investigations/ Diagnosis

Histopathology. Differentiate from other causes of lumps or ulcers, particularly:
- lip salivary tumours—from mucocele
- tongue salivary tumours—from carcinoma
- palatal salivary tumours—from oral carcinoma, antral carcinoma or necrotizing sialometaplasia.

Treatment

Excision and microscopic examination (see p. 143).

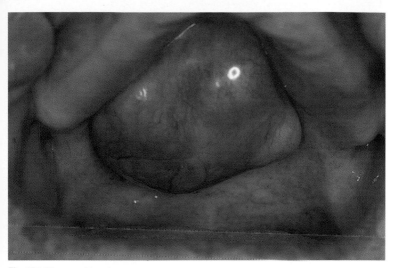

Fig. 106 Pleomorphic adenoma.

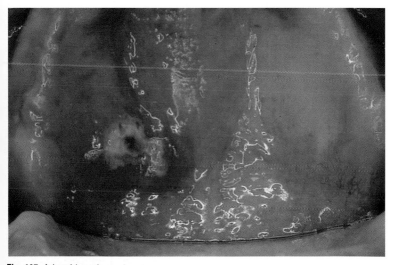

Fig. 107 Adenoid cystic carcinoma.

Mucocele

*Incidence/
Aetiology*

Common. Usually extravasation of mucus from damaged duct; rarely retention of mucus within salivary gland or its duct (see also p. 21).

Clinical features

Mucoceles are dome-shaped, bluish, translucent, fluctuant, painless, and rupture easily. Recur frequently. Deeper mucoceles are less common and are often retention cysts. *Ranula* 'frog belly' is a large mucocele in the floor of the mouth (Fig. 108). May involve the sublingual gland or, rarely, burrow through mylohyoid (plunging ranula).
   Superficial mucoceles are rare small intra-epithelial lesions simulating a vesiculobullous disorder.

*Investigations/
Diagnosis*

Microscopic features. Diagnosis is clearcut but neoplasm must be excluded, particularly in the *upper* lip (see p. 99).

Treatment

If asymptomatic and small, observe; otherwise, use cryosurgery or excision including gland.

Salivary duct obstruction

*Incidence/
Aetiology*

Fairly common. Usually calculus in submandibular duct (see also page 137).

Clinical features

Pain and swelling at meals (Fig. 109). Stone may or may not be palpable.

*Investigations/
Diagnosis*

Plain radiographs ± sialography. Differentiate from stricture or neoplasm.

Treatment

Usually incise duct and remove stone.

Dermoid cyst

*Incidence/
Aetiology*

Developmental; rare.

Clinical features

Doughy painless swelling in midline floor of mouth (Fig. 110).

*Investigations/
Diagnosis*

Aspirate. Differentiate from ranula or cystic hygroma.

Treatment

Remove surgically.

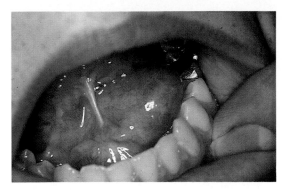

Fig. 108 Ranula.

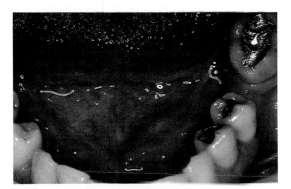

Fig. 109 Obstruction of submandibular duct.

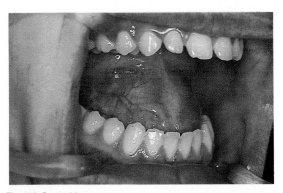

Fig. 110 Dermoid cyst.

Langerhans cell histiocytoses (Histiocytosis X)

This term includes:
- solitary eosinophilic granuloma of bone
- multifocal eosinophilic granuloma (Hand–Schüller–Christian disease)
- Letterer–Siwe disease.

Incidence/ Aetiology

Rare: male predilection. Neoplasms arising from Langerhans cells (dendritic intraepithelial antigen-presenting cells). NB. *Not* granulomas histologically.

Clinical features

Solitary eosinophilic granuloma: usually benign with osteolytic lesion only. It is mainly seen in adults. There is sometimes gross periodontal destruction (Fig. 111).

Multifocal eosinophilic granuloma: Hand–Schüller–Christian disease—more malignant form in children and young adults characterized by osteolytic lesions and sometimes diabetes insipidus and proptosis.

Letterer–Siwe disease: most malignant form in infants characterized by failure to thrive, fever, hepatosplenomegaly, and skeletal osteolytic lesions that may affect the jaws with pain, swelling and loosening of teeth.

Investigations/ Diagnosis

Biopsy: foamy macrophages (Birbeck granules may be seen by EM), eosinophils and bone destruction. Differentiate from other osteolytic disorders, especially carcinomatosis and myelomatosis.

Treatment

Surgery for solitary lesions; radiotherapy/ chemotherapy for multifocal disease.

Granulomatous diseases

Crohn's disease (see pp. 17 & 47; Figs 112 & 113).

Sarcoidosis (see pp. 17 & 137).

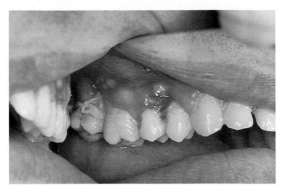

Fig. 111 Langerhans cell histiocytosis.

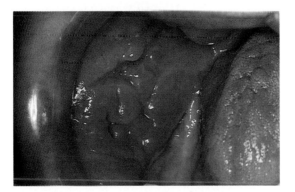

Fig. 112 Crohn's disease: cobble-stoning of buccal mucosa.

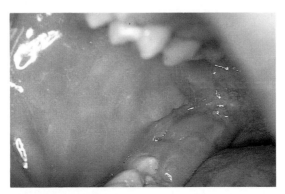

Fig. 113 Crohn's disease: mucosal tags.

Torus palatinus and torus mandibularis

Incidence/ Aetiology

Genetic; usually in adults, especially females. Common in Mongoloid races.

Clinical features

Torus palatinus: slow-growing, asymptomatic, bony lump in midline of palate (Fig. 114).

Torus mandibularis: bilateral asymptomatic bony lumps lingual to premolars (Fig. 115).

Investigations/ Diagnosis

Radiography—but usually clinically obvious. Torus palatinus—neoplasms should be excluded. Torus mandibularis—exclude unerupted teeth.

Treatment

Nil. Excise or reduce only if causing severe difficulties, e.g. with dentures.

Gardner syndrome

This condition presents with jaw osteomas (Fig. 116), polyposis coli, epidermoid cysts, desmoid tumours and pigmented lesions of fundus of eye.

Paget's disease

Incidence/ Aetiology

Unknown: virus has been implicated—possibly measles or respiratory syncytial virus. Common, with up to 5% of those affected over 55 years of age.

Clinical features

Progressive jaw swelling: hypercementosis.

Investigations/ Diagnosis

Radiography; raised serum alkaline phosphatase and urinary hydroxyproline. Differentiate from bone neoplasms.

Treatment

Bisphosphonates or calcitonin.

Fibrous dysplasia

Incidence/ Aetiology

Unknown. Rare, usually appearing in childhood.

Clinical features

Painless swelling of jaw.

Investigations/ Diagnosis

Radiography; biopsy; raised serum alkaline phosphatase. Differentiate from bone neoplasms.

Treatment

Cosmetic surgery. Typically self-limiting.

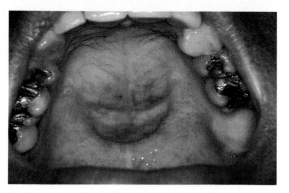

Fig. 114 Torus palatinus.

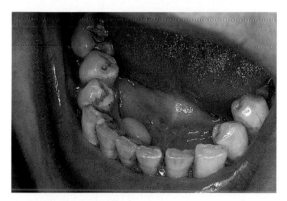

Fig. 115 Torus mandibularis.

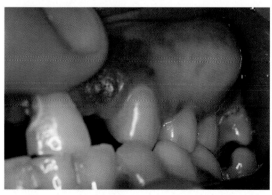

Fig. 116 Gardner syndrome.

Ankyloglossia (tongue-tie)

Incidence/
Aetiology

Rare, especially complete or lateral ankyloglossia. Most cases are partial. May be genetic basis.

Clinical features

Lingual fraenum anchors tongue tip, restricting protrusion and lateral movements (Fig. 117). Oral cleansing (but not speech) is impaired.

Diagnosis

Differentiate from tethering of tongue by scarring in epidermolysis bullosa (see p. 53). Tongue-tie is also seen in some rare syndromes.

Treatment

Surgery if severe.

Macroglossia

Incidence/
Aetiology

Uncommon.

Congenital: lymphangioma (see p. 93); haemangioma (see pp. 75 & 111); neurofibromatosis (see p. 111); Down syndrome; cretinism; Hurler syndrome.

Acquired: acromegaly; amyloidosis (see p. 109).

Clinical features

Tongue indented by teeth, or too large to be contained in the mouth (Fig. 118). Haemangioma gives it a purplish colour (see Fig. 122, p. 112).

Diagnosis

Biopsy, but not if angiomatous.

Treatment

Observe, or surgically reduce (but see p. 109).

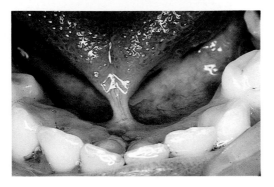

Fig. 117 Ankyloglossia.

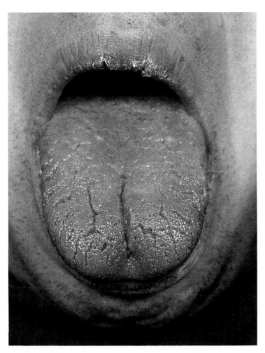

Fig. 118 Macroglossia and cheilitis in Down syndrome.

Amyloidosis

Incidence/ Aetiology

Rare. Deposition in tissues of eosinophilic hyaline material, with a fibrillar structure on ultramicroscopy.

Deposits are immunoglobulin light chains in primary (usually myeloma-associated or other monoclonal gammopathy) amyloid.

Different proteins (AA proteins) are present in secondary and other forms of amyloid. Secondary amyloidosis is now seen mainly in rheumatoid arthritis and ulcerative colitis, and rarely affects the mouth.

Clinical features

Oral amyloidosis is almost exclusively primary. Macroglossia, in up to 50% of patients (Figs 119 & 120), and oral petechiae or blood-filled bullae (secondary purpura).

Investigations/ Diagnosis

Biopsy; blood picture; ESR and marrow biopsy; serum proteins and electrophoresis; urinalysis (Bence–Jones proteinuria); skeletal survey for myeloma. Differentiate from other causes of macroglossia (see p. 107), and from other causes of petechiae/bullae, such as localized oral purpura and bleeding tendency.

Treatment

Chemotherapy with melphalan, corticosteroids or fluoxymesterone.

Surgical reduction of the tongue is inadvisable; tissue is friable, often bleeds excessively and swelling quickly recurs.

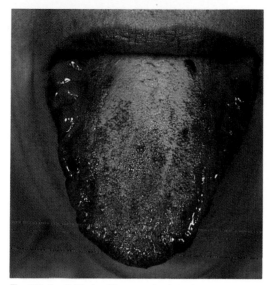

Fig. 119 Amyloidosis with macroglossia and purpura.

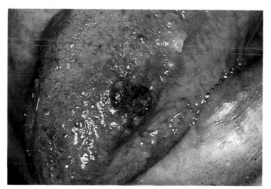

Fig. 120 Amyloidosis showing macroglossia and purpura.

Neurilemmoma (schwannoma)

Incidence/Aetiology

Rare benign neoplasm of neurilemmal cells of axonal sheath.

Clinical features

Slowly enlarging painless mass, usually in tongue. Multiple neurilemmomas can sometimes be found in von Recklinghausen's neurofibromatosis.

Investigations/Diagnosis

Histopathology. Differentiate from any other soft tissue tumour.

Treatment

Excision and microscopic examination.

Neurofibroma

Incidence/Aetiology

Rare benign tumour arising from specialized fibroblasts of neural sheath.

Clinical features

Painless slow-growing soft mass, usually in the tongue (Fig. 121). Multiple neurofibromas characteristic of von Recklinghausen's neurofibromatosis are present, but are more common in skin with *café au lait* hyperpigmentation, than in the mouth. Macroglossia and bone hypertrophy are rarely present. Neurofibromas occasionally undergo sarcomatous change.

Mucosal 'neurofibromas' (plexiform neuromas) may be seen in multiple endocrine neoplasia type III syndrome (with medullary carcinoma of the thyroid).

Investigations/Diagnosis

Biopsy. Not clinically distinguishable from other benign soft tissue tumours.

Treatment

Excision and microscopy; general examination for neurofibromatosis and skin pigmentation.

Haemangioma

See page 75 and Figure 122.

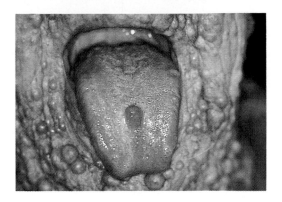

Fig. 121 Neurofibroma of tongue in von Recklinghausen's neurofibromatosis.

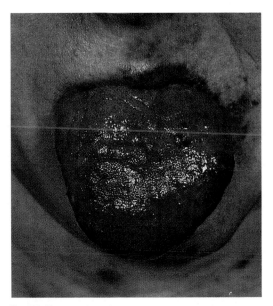

Fig. 122 Haemangioma involving tongue causing macroglossia.

Fissured (scrotal) tongue

Incidence/ Aetiology

Common. Often hereditary. A fissured tongue is found in many normal persons, often in Down syndrome and in Melkersson–Rosenthal syndrome.

Clinical features

Multiple fissures; commonly associated with erythema migrans (Fig. 123). The condition is of no consequence. Sometimes the tongue is sore for no apparent reason.

Investigations/ Diagnosis

None, but blood picture if tongue is sore. The diagnosis is usually clearcut. Lobulated tongue of Sjögren syndrome and chronic mucocutaneous candidosis must be differentiated.

Treatment

Nil; reassure.

Erythema migrans (benign migratory glossitis; geographic tongue)

Incidence/ Aetiology

Common. Genetic. 1–2% of adults. Also seen in infancy. Associated with psoriasis in 4%.

Clinical features

Often asymptomatic, occasionally sore, especially with acidic foods (e.g. tomatoes). There are irregular, pink or red depapillated areas, sometimes surrounded by distinct yellowish slightly raised margins (Fig. 124). Red areas change in shape, increase in size, and spread or move to other areas within hours. Typically involves the dorsum of the tongue, rarely adjacent oral mucosa. The tongue is often also fissured.

Investigations/ Diagnosis

History of migrating pattern. Similar lesions may be seen in psoriasis, and Reiter syndrome (transiently). There also may be confusion with lichen planus and lupus erythematosus.

Treatment

Reassure.

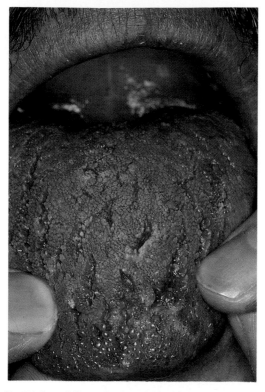

Fig. 123 Scrotal (fissured) tongue (also shows some erythema migrans).

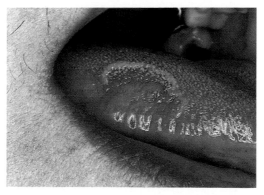

Fig. 124 Geographic tongue (erythema migrans or benign migratory glossitis).

Deficiency glossitis

*Incidence/
Aetiology*

Uncommon except in malabsorption states, pernicious anaemia or the occasional vegan or other dietary faddist. Deficiencies of iron, folic acid, vitamin B_{12} (rarely other B vitamins) can cause sore tongue which may appear normal, or may be red and depapillated.

Clinical features

Tongue may appear completely normal, or there may be linear or patchy red lesions (especially in vitamin B_{12} deficiency, Fig. 125), depapillation with erythema (in deficiencies of iron, folic acid or B vitamins) or pallor (iron deficiency). Lingual depapillation begins at the tip and margins of the dorsum but later involves the whole dorsum (Fig. 126). Various patterns are described. There may also be oral ulceration (see p. 25) and angular stomatitis (see p. 11).

Rare types of deficiency glossitis include:
- Riboflavin: papillae enlarge initially but are later lost
- Niacin: red, swollen, enlarged 'beefy' tongue
- Pyridoxine: swollen, purplish tongue.

*Investigations/
Diagnosis*

Blood picture. Vitamin assays or biopsy are rarely indicated. Differentiate from erythema migrans, lichen planus and acute candidosis.

Treatment

Replacement therapy *after underlying cause of deficiency established and rectified.*

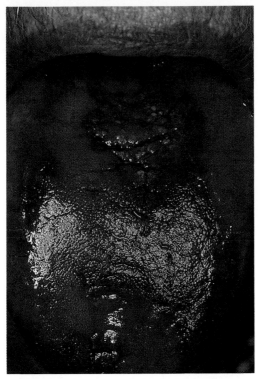

Fig. 125 Glossitis in deficiency of vitamin B$_{12}$ (pernicious anaemia) showing patchy erythema but minimal depapillation.

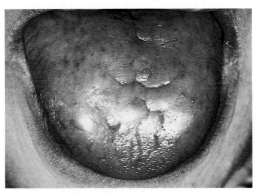

Fig. 126 Atrophic glossitis.

Median rhomboid glossitis

Incidence/
Aetiology

Uncommon. It is seen mainly in adult males who smoke. Possibly a congenital anomaly but rarely seen before middle age. It may be acquired, and is sometimes infected with *Candida* species. Similar lesions may be seen in HIV infection.

Clinical features

May be rhomboidal (diamond-shaped) red, or nodular and depapillated or white, in midline of dorsum of tongue, just anterior to circumvallate papillae (Fig. 127).

Investigation/
Diagnosis

Smear and Gram stain for *Candida albicans*. Biopsy is rarely required (can show pseudoepitheliomatous hyperplasia). Differentiate from erythema migrans, erythroplasia and carcinoma (see above).

Treatment

Antifungals if candidal; stop smoking.

Candidal glossitis

Incidence/
Aetiology

Uncommon except in above groups. Opportunistic infection with candida species, particularly *C. albicans*. Predisposing factors include: broad spectrum antimicrobials, particularly tetracycline; xerostomia; topical corticosteroids (more often thrush); immune defect (more often thrush).

Clinical features

Diffuse erythema and soreness (Fig. 128). There may also be patches of thrush (see p. 59), particularly in upper buccal sulcus posteriorly.

Investigations/
Diagnosis

Smear for candidal hyphae. Differentiate from deficiency glossitis.

Treatment

Treat predisposing cause; antifungals (see p. 59).

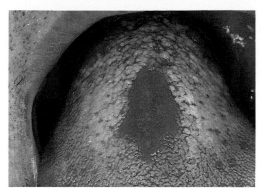

Fig. 127 Median rhomboid glossitis.

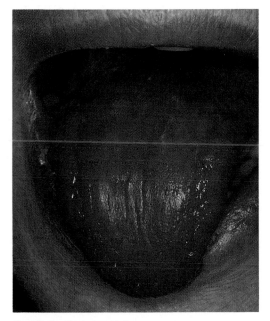

Fig. 128 Candidal glossitis in xerostomia.

Sjögren syndrome

Clinical features

Xerostomia in Sjögren syndrome predisposes to depapillated lobulated tongue and candidosis. Sore tongue is lobulated (not merely fissured) in quilt-like fashion and often diffusely erythematous as a result of candidosis (Fig. 129).

Investigations/ Diagnosis

Differentiate from deficiency states and other causes of xerostomia, especially:
- drugs (anticholinergics, especially tricyclic antidepressants and sympathomimetics)
- dehydration
- salivary gland disease: irradiation
- sarcoidosis (see p. 137).

Treatment

Sialogogues or artificial saliva; antifungals.

'Burning mouth' (oral dysaesthesia)

Incidence/ Aetiology

Common, especially in middle-aged females. Several predisposing factors include organic lesions, e.g. deficiency states, erythema migrans, ulcers (see p. 23), lichen planus and candidosis. A normal-appearing tongue is present in deficiency states, and with psychogenic causes, drugs (e.g. captopril) and diabetes mellitus. This section deals only with a normal but sore tongue.

Clinical features

Almost invariably persistent burning sensation in tongue (occasionally in palate) with no organic disease (Fig. 130). Few profess anxiety about cancer or sexually transmitted disease; some admit this on specific questioning.

Investigations/ Diagnosis

Blood picture to exclude organic causes; psychiatric investigation for depression. Differentiate from organic causes outlined above.

Treatment

Treat any organic cause. Otherwise, cognitive therapy or antidepressants (usually prothiaden). B vitamins are rarely helpful.

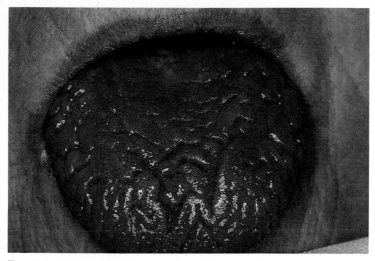

Fig. 129 Lobulated tongue typical of advanced Sjögren syndrome.

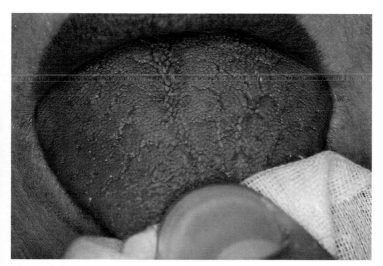

Fig. 130 Burning mouth syndrome: normal appearance of tongue in this syndrome which often has a psychogenic basis.

Furred tongue

*Incidence/
Aetiology*

Common in febrile illnesses. Often unknown cause, but sometimes poor oral hygiene, infections (Fig. 131), dehydration or soft diet. Debris and bacteria accumulate, especially if diet contains little roughage. An upper denture also does not clean the tongue as effectively as palatal rugae.

Clinical features

The tongue has yellowish 'fur' which may be discoloured by foods or drugs.

Diagnosis

Exclusion of the following differential diagnoses: thrush (rarely on dorsum of tongue), chronic candidosis, hairy leukoplakia (lateral borders of tongue) or other leukoplakias.

Treatment

Treat underlying condition.

Black or brown hairy tongue

*Incidence/
Aetiology*

Uncommon: mainly in middle aged or older males. Unknown aetiology. Smoking, drugs (e.g. iron salts, griseofulvin) and poor oral hygiene (proliferation of chromogenic microorganisms, not *Candida albicans*) may predispose.

Clinical features

Brown or black hairy appearance of central dorsum of tongue, most severe posteriorly (Fig. 132).

Diagnosis

Diagnosis clinical.

Treatment

Improve oral hygiene; discontinue any drugs responsible; brush tongue (in evenings); suck pineapple or dry peach stone (yes!); apply retinoic acid.

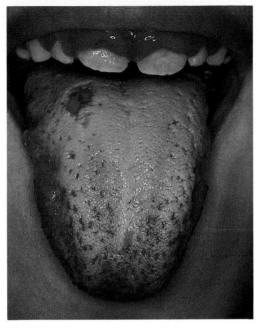

Fig. 131 Furred tongue: common in febrile illnesses (herpetic stomatitis in this case).

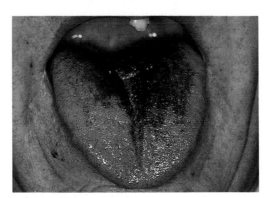

Fig. 132 Black hairy tongue.

Chronic marginal gingivitis

Incidence/ Aetiology

Almost universal in adults to some degree. Dental bacterial plaque.

Clinical features

Erythema, oedema and painless swelling of marginal gingivae with bleeding on brushing or eating hard foods (Fig. 133).

Investigations/ Diagnosis

Usually clinically obvious; radiography. Differentiate from desquamative gingivitis (p. 133).

Treatment

Oral hygiene, including scaling; root-planing, etc., if periodontitis associated.

Pregnancy gingivitis and epulis

Incidence/ Aetiology

Common. Exacerbation of chronic gingivitis mainly after 2nd month of pregnancy.

Clinical features

Pregnancy gingivitis: erythema, swelling and liability to bleed (Fig. 134).

Pregnancy epulis: Occasionally, a proliferative response leads to pregnancy epulis (pyogenic granuloma). Soft, red or occasionally firm, swelling of dental papilla anteriorly (Fig. 135). It may be asymptomatic unless traumatized by biting or toothbrushing.

Investigations/ Diagnosis

Biopsy rarely. Pregnancy test occasionally.

Pregnancy gingivitis: differentiate from Wegener's granulomatosis.

Pregnancy epulis: differentiate from other epulides.

Treatment

Pregnancy gingivitis: oral hygiene.

Pregnancy epulis: oral hygiene. If asymptomatic, leave alone—may regress after parturition. If symptomatic, excision biopsy.

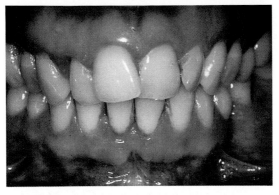

Fig. 133 Chronic marginal gingivitis: erythema, swelling of marginal gingiva and papillae.

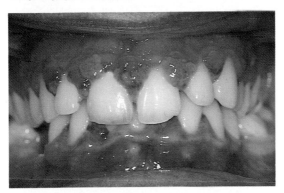

Fig. 134 Pregnancy gingivitis (if proliferative, resembles Wegener's granulomatosis as here).

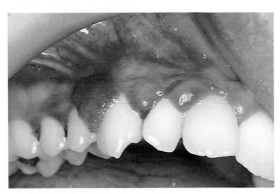

Fig. 135 Pregnancy epulis.

Generalized gingival swelling

Incidence/
Aetiology
Common in mouthbreathers. Other causes include the following:

Congenital
- Hereditary gingival fibromatosis (Fig. 136): usually then in isolation, occasionally as part of a wider syndrome.
- Mucopolysaccharidoses and mucolipidoses.

Acquired
- Chronic oedematous gingivitis in mouthbreathers with poor oral hygiene.
- Drugs: phenytoin, cyclosporin, or calcium channel blockers (Figs 137 & 138).
- Leukaemia (see p. 127).
- Scurvy (see p. 127).
- Chronic granulomas: Crohn's disease and sarcoidosis (see p. 129).
- Wegener's granulomatosis (see p. 129).

Clinical features
Drug-induced hyperplasia is usually aggravated by poor oral hygiene, and starts interdentally, especially labially. Papillae firm, pale and enlarge to form false vertical clefts (Figs 137 & 138). This is associated with hypertrichosis in congenital and drug-induced types. In others, the clinical features depend on the aetiology.

Investigations/
Diagnosis
Various, as appropriate. Blood picture in some cases; biopsy occasionally.

Treatment
Treat predisposing factors; improve oral hygiene; gingivoplasty where indicated.

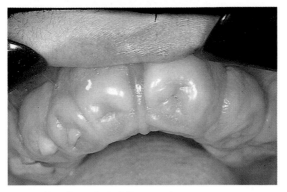

Fig. 136 Hereditary gingival fibromatosis.

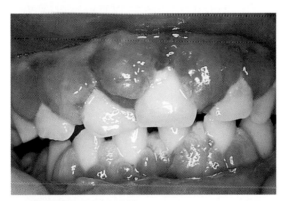

Fig. 137 Phenytoin hyperplasia.

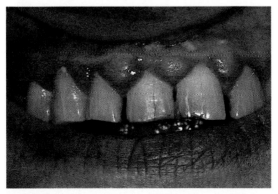

Fig. 138 Calcium channel blocker (nifedipine) hyperplasia.

Scurvy

Incidence/
Aetiology

Clinical curiosity now. Absence of fresh fruit or vegetables for long periods leads to vitamin C (ascorbic acid) deficiency.

Clinical features

Gingivae: diffusely swollen, boggy, and purplish with purpura and haemorrhage (Fig. 139).

Skin: perifollicular haemorrhages.

Investigations/
Diagnosis

Dietary history; clinical features; white cell ascorbic acid. Differentiate from leukaemia particularly.

Treatment

Vitamin C supplements; reform diet.

Leukaemia

Gingival involvement in leukaemia is most common in adults and is characterized by swelling haemorrhage and ulceration (Figs 140 & 141). Gingival swelling is most characteristic of acute myelomonocytic leukaemia. Petechiae, ecchymoses or haemorrhage are common and ulceration may develop (see also pp. 7 & 43).

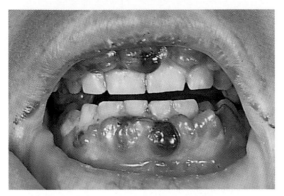

Fig. 139 Scurvy: gingival swelling and haemorrhage.

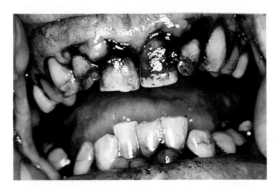

Fig. 140 Leukaemia: spontaneous gingival haemorrhage and purpura.

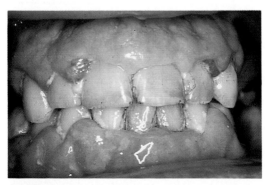

Fig. 141 Leukaemia: gingival swelling (a feature particularly of myelomonocytic leukaemia).

Epulides

Epulides are localized gingival swellings and rarely true neoplasms.

Aetiology

Fibrous epulides: may result from local gingival irritation, leading to fibrous hyperplasia (Fig. 142).

Pyogenic granulomas: (see p. 5) uncommon except as pregnancy epulides (lesions themselves not histologically distinguishable) (Fig. 143).

Giant cell epulides: may result from proliferation of giant cells persisting after resorption of deciduous teeth. Rarely, epulides are metastatic carcinomas or other tumours.

Clinical features

Fibrous epulides are most common; they typically form narrow, firm, pale swellings of an anterior interdental papilla and may ulcerate. Giant cell/pregnancy/neoplastic epulides are soft, deeper red but cannot be distinguished from fibrous epulides clinically with certainty.

Investigations/ Diagnosis

Excision biopsy; radiography.

Treatment

Excision; remove local irritants (calculus).

Other gingival hyperplasias

Crohn's disease: see pages 17 & 47.

Sarcoidosis: see pages 17 & 137.

Malignant diseases
- *Carcinoma of the gingiva* is uncommon (Fig. 144).
- *Secondary deposits* are rare, but can mimic 'simple' epulides.
- *Kaposi's sarcoma* occasionally affects gingiva in AIDS (see p. 79).
- *Histiocytosis X* may cause gingival ulceration and destruction of periodontium rather than hyperplasia (see p. 103).

Wegener's granulomatosis can present an almost pathognomonic 'strawberry' appearance of gingiva. There may be lung and kidney lesions, and serum anti-neutrophil cytoplasmic antibodies (ANCA). Chemotherapy or co-trimoxazole are indicated.

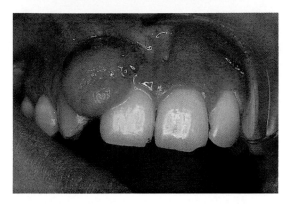

Fig. 142 Fibrous epulis (compare with pregnancy epulis, Fig. 135).

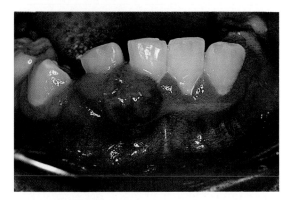

Fig. 143 Pyogenic granuloma.

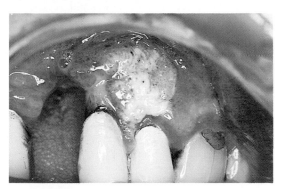

Fig. 144 Carcinoma of gingiva.

Infections

A few infections may cause gingival lesions. Herpetic stomatitis and acute ulcerative (necrotizing) gingivitis have characteristic clinical pictures.

Herpetic stomatitis

Gingivae are typically swollen, boggy and purplish (Figs 131 & 145) occasionally with vesicles and ulcers (Fig. 146) (see also p. 29).

Acute ulcerative gingivitis

Incidence/ Aetiology

Uncommon except in lower socioeconomic groups. Typically an infection of adolescents and young adults, especially in institutions, armed forces, etc. Non-contagious anaerobic infection associated with overwhelming proliferation of *Borrelia vincentii* and fusiform bacteria. Predisposing factors include smoking, viral respiratory infections and immune defects such as in HIV/AIDS (see also p. 37).

Clinical features

Characteristic features are severe soreness, profuse gingival bleeding, halitosis and a bad taste. Interdental papillae ulcerated with necrotic slough and unpleasant halitosis (Figs 147 & 42, p. 38). Malaise, fever and/or cervical lymphadenitis (unlike herpetic stomatitis) are rare. Cancrum oris (noma) is a very rare complication, usually in debilitated children.

Investigations/ Diagnosis

Smear for fusospirochaetal bacteria and leucocytes; blood picture occasionally. Diagnosis usually clearcut, but occasionally there may be confusion with acute leukaemia or herpetic stomatitis.

Treatment

Oral debridement; metronidazole (penicillin if pregnant); oral hygiene.

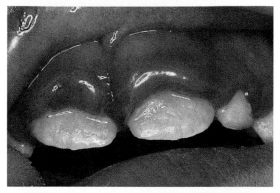

Fig. 145 Primary herpetic stomatitis: diffuse swollen, boggy, purple gingiva, and ulcers.

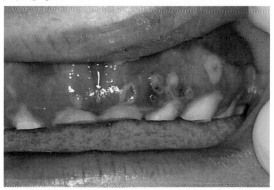

Fig. 146 Primary herpetic stomatitis (ulcers are more prominent in this patient).

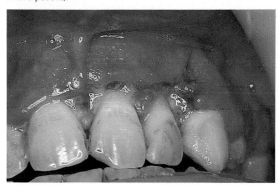

Fig. 147 Acute ulcerative gingivitis: recognized complication of HIV infection.

'Desquamative gingivitis'

Not a disease entity but a clinical term for persistently sore, glazed and red or ulcerated gingivae (see also pp. 51 & 57).

Incidence/
Aetiology

Usually a manifestation of atrophic lichen planus or mucous membrane pemphigoid. Occasionally seen in pemphigus or other dermatoses (dermatitis herpetiformis, linear IgA disease), or drugs/chemicals (sodium lauryl sulphate).
   Fairly common. It is almost exclusively a disease of middle-aged or elderly females.

Clinical features

Gingivae are red and glazed, patchily or uniformly, especially labially (Figs 56, p. 50, 148 & 149). Gingival margins and edentulous ridges tend to be spared. Erythema is exaggerated where oral hygiene is poor. Other oral or cutaneous lesions of dermatoses may be associated.

Investigations/
Diagnosis

Biopsy. Differentiate mainly from acute candidosis and chronic marginal gingivitis (p. 123).

Treatment

Improve oral hygiene; topical corticosteroids, or dapsone. Corticosteroid creams used overnight in a polythene splint may help.

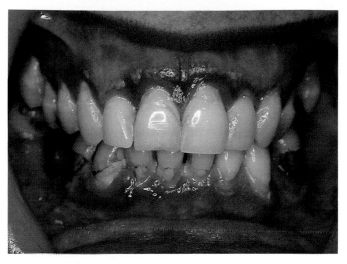

Fig. 148 Desquamative gingivitis due to lichen planus.

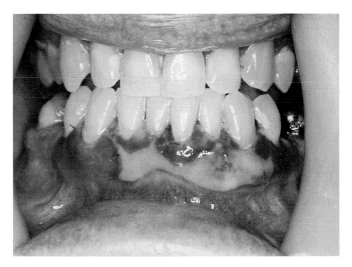

Fig. 149 Desquamative gingivitis due to mucous membrane pemphigoid.

Mumps (acute viral parotitis)

Incidence/Aetiology

Fairly common; typically in children. Mumps virus; rarely Coxsackie, ECHO, EBV or HIV infection.

Clinical features

Incubation period 14–21 days. Often subclinical. Malaise, fever, anorexia and sialadenitis. Painful, diffuse swelling of one/both parotids and sometimes submandibular glands (Fig. 150). Saliva is non-purulent; the duct is inflamed. Also trismus and dry mouth are present. Complications are uncommon but include pancreatitis, encephalitis, orchitis, oophoritis and deafness.

Investigations/Diagnosis

Mumps antibody titres (rarely needed); serum amylases or lipases (occasionally). Differentiate from obstructive and/or bacterial sialadenitis mainly (see below and p. 137).

Treatment

Symptomatic.

Acute bacterial (ascending) parotitis

Incidence/Aetiology

Rare, except in association with xerostomia. Usually the infection ascends the duct of a non-functioning gland. Infectious agents include pneumococci, *Staphylococcus aureus* or viridans streptococci.

Clinical features

Painful swelling of one gland only, with red, shiny overlying skin, trismus, and purulent discharge from duct (Fig. 151).

Investigations/Diagnosis

Pus for culture and sensitivities. Differentiate mainly from mumps (above and see p. 137).

Treatment

Antimicrobials (flucloxacillin if staphylococcal and not allergic to penicillin); sialogogues.

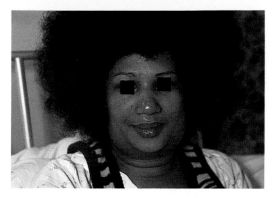

Fig. 150 Mumps: bilateral swellings of parotid and submandibular salivary glands in this patient.

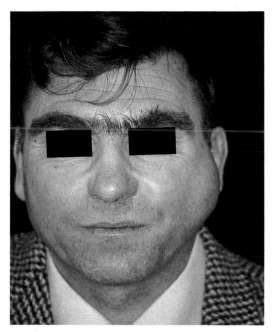

Fig. 151 Acute bacterial parotitis.

Salivary obstruction

Incidence/
Aetiology

Fairly common in submandibular duct or gland. Calculus usually; rarely mucus plug, fibrous stricture or neoplasm (see also p. 101).

Clinical features

May be asymptomatic. Typically pain and swelling of gland at meals (Fig. 152). Obstruction of minor salivary gland duct may produce a mucocele (see pp. 21 & 101).

Investigations/
Diagnosis

Radiography (but 40% of stones are radiolucent); sialography if necessary. Differentiate from other causes of salivary swelling: inflammatory—mumps, bacterial sialadenitis, Sjögren syndrome, sarcoidosis; duct obstruction; neoplasms (see p. 141); others including sialosis, drugs and Mikulicz disease.

Treatment

Surgical removal of obstruction $\pm$ lithotripsy for calculus.

Sarcoidosis

Incidence/
Aetiology

Uncommon. Unknown cause.

Clinical features

Salivary gland swelling usually painless, bilateral (Fig. 153). Often with xerostomia. Rarely: fever, uveitis and facial palsy (uveoparotid fever: Heerfordt syndrome). Other features include erythema nodosum and lung involvement (see also pp. 17 & 129).

Investigations/
Diagnosis

Biopsy; chest radiograph; Kveim test; gallium scan, raised serum angiotensin converting enzyme (SACE) and adenosine deaminase. Differentiate from other causes of salivary gland swelling (particularly sialosis and Sjögren syndrome: see p. 139) and from xerostomia (see p. 139).

Treatment

Corticosteroids if lung or eye involvement, or hypercalcaemia.

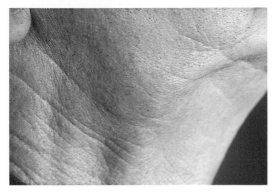

Fig. 152 Swelling of submandibular salivary gland caused by ductal obstruction by a stone.

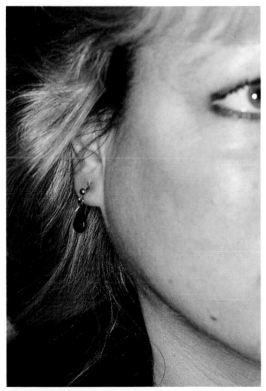

Fig. 153 Sarcoidosis: parotid salivary gland swelling.

Sjögren syndrome

Incidence/
Aetiology

Uncommon: mainly middle-aged or elderly women. Autoimmune inflammatory exocrinopathy.

Clinical features

Dry eyes (keratoconjunctivitis sicca): initially asymptomatic, later gritty sensation, itching, soreness or inability to cry. Salivary and lacrimal glands may swell (Fig. 154). Dry mouth (xerostomia): difficulty in eating dry foods, disturbed taste, speech and swallowing, rampant caries, candidosis and acute sialadenitis. Saliva is frothy and not pooling; parchment-like mucosa (Fig. 155) and lobulated depapillated tongue. Uncommon complication is lymphoma. There is no connective tissue disease in primary, but present in secondary Sjögren syndrome: typically rheumatoid arthritis or primary biliary cirrhosis, and occasionally other autoimmune disorders. Dry mouth and/or salivary swelling may also be seen in HIV disease.

Investigations/
Diagnosis

Salivary flow rates are reduced. Labial gland biopsy; sialography and/or scintigraphy; auto-antibodies, especially rheumatoid factor, Ro (SS-A) and La (SS-B) (not in HIV disease). Exclude other causes (see p. 141).

Treatment

Control underlying disease: at present experimental (e.g. cyclosporin).
- Eyes—methylcellulose eye drops or rarely ligation or cautery of nasolacrimal duct.
- Dry mouth—preventive dental care (oral hygiene, limitation of sucrose intake, fluorides, chlorhexidine).
- Treat infection.
- Sialogogues and/or salivary substitutes (e.g. methylcellulose). Pilocarpine or bethanecol may be used to stimulate salivation.

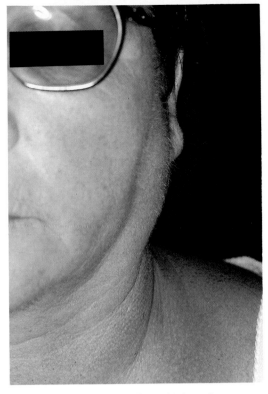

Fig. 154 Sjögren syndrome: salivary glands swell at some stage in about a third of patients.

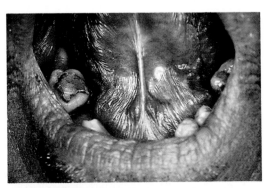

Fig. 155 Sjögren syndrome: severe xerostomia.

Dry mouth

Incidence/
Aetiology

A common subjective complaint: objective evidence less common.
The main causes include:

Iatrogenic
- Drugs, such as tricyclics, lithium, phenothiazines anti-retroviral agents and antihistamines.
- Irradiation of major salivary glands.
- Rarely—cytotoxic agents or graft versus host disease.

Non-iatrogenic
- Uncontrolled diabetes.
- Sjögren syndrome (see p. 139).
- Sarcoidosis (see p. 17).
- HIV disease (see p. 159).
  Sequelae of dry mouth include: caries (Fig. 156), candidosis and ascending sialadenitis.

Sialosis

Incidence/
Aetiology

Uncommon. Frequently 'idiopathic'. Known causes include:

Neurogenic: various drugs such as isoprenaline.

Dystrophic-metabolic: anorexia-bulimia, alcoholic cirrhosis, diabetes, malnutrition, thyroid disease, acromegaly and pregnancy.
Common feature is autonomic dysfunction.

Clinical features

Painless bilateral swelling, typically of parotids (Fig. 157).

*Investigations/
Diagnosis*

Blood glucose; liver function tests; possibly growth hormone levels.

Treatment

Exclude and treat predisposing cause.

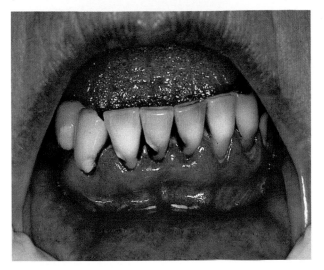

Fig. 156 Dental caries: sequel of dry mouth.

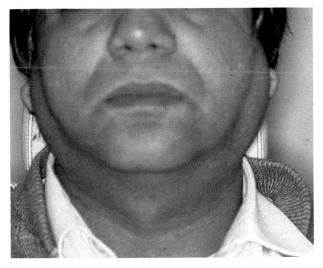

Fig. 157 Sialosis: bilateral swelling of parotids.

Salivary gland neoplasms

Classification of salivary neoplasms:
- Adenomas
  — Pleomorphic
  — Monomorphic: adenolymphoma/oncocytic adenoma/others
- Mucoepidermoid carcinoma
- Acinic cell carcinoma
- Adenoid cystic and other carcinomas.

Incidence/ Aetiology

Rare: mainly in middle and old age. Irradiation and viruses, such as EBV, implicated in some human neoplasms (see also pp. 97 and 99).

Clinical features

Typically cause asymptomatic swelling in one gland (usually parotid) and eversion of ear lobe (Fig. 158). No xerostomia. Malignant neoplasms classically (Fig. 159) grow rapidly, cause pain, may ulcerate, and may involve nerves (e.g. facial palsy).

General features: 75% involve parotid; 60% are pleomorphic salivary adenomas and benign. Most tumours in sublingual gland are malignant. 46% in minor salivary glands and 18% in major are malignant.

Investigations/ Diagnosis

Microscopy after parotidectomy (biopsy allows seeding and recurrence). Differentiate from non-neoplastic salivary gland swellings.

Treatment

Surgical excision; radiotherapy also for some.

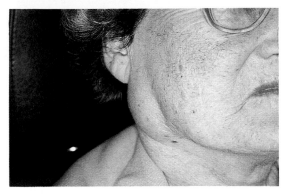

Fig. 158 Pleomorphic adenoma of parotid.

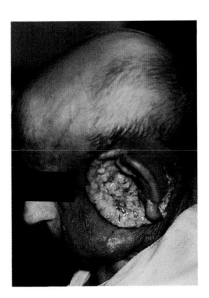

Fig. 159 Extensive ulcerated
adenocarcinoma of parotid.

9 / Cervical lymph node swellings

Incidence/
Aetiology

Common.

Inflammatory causes
Infection   (the usual cause)
- Local viral or bacterial (dental, scalp, ear, nose or throat): including cat-scratch disease and staphylococcal lymphadenitis.
- Systemic: viral, e.g. infectious mononucleosis, cytomegalovirus, or HIV infection; bacterial, including syphilis, tuberculosis, non-tuberculous mycobacterioses; brucellosis; fungal (rarely); parasitic, toxoplasmosis; Kawasaki disease (mucocutaneous lymph node syndrome).

Others: sarcoid, connective tissue diseases.

Malignant causes
Local: oral, scalp, ear, nose or throat usually; rarely thyroid.

Systemic: leukaemias and lymphomas, carcinomas, Letterer–Siwe disease.

Drugs
Particularly phenytoin.

Clinical features

Lymphadenitis: discrete tender, mobile, enlarged firm nodes (Fig. 160); rarely suppurate.

Metastases: discrete or matted, fixed, enlarged, hard nodes (rubbery in lymphomas); may ulcerate.

Investigations/
Diagnosis

Search for lesion in drainage area; blood picture; biopsy if neoplasm suspected.

Treatment

Treat cause (above).

Actinomycosis

Rare bacterial infection below mandibular angle (not lymph nodes) that may rarely follow jaw fracture or tooth extraction (Fig. 161). Prolonged, therapy, usually with penicillin, is indicated.

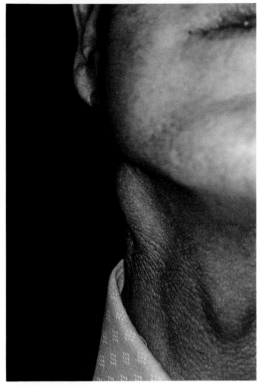

Fig. 160 Tuberculous lymphadenitis.

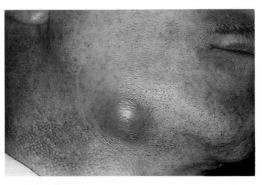

Fig. 161 Actinomycosis.

Facial palsy

Incidence

Uncommon. Usually stroke or Bell's palsy.

Clinical features

Upper motor neurone lesions (e.g. stroke): unilateral palsy mainly in lower face; may be features of stroke but hearing or taste normal.

Lower motor neurone lesions (e.g. Bell's palsy): complete unilateral facial palsy; may be loss of taste and/or hyperacusis (Figs 162 & 163).

Investigations/ Diagnosis

Neurological; blood pressure. Differentiate from inflammatory, traumatic and neoplastic lesions. Lyme disease (in some areas), diabetes and HIV are occasional causes.

Treatment

Bell's palsy: systemic corticosteroids.

Trigeminal neuralgia

Incidence/ Aetiology

Uncommon; mainly in middle and old age. Aetiology unclear.

Clinical features

Pain is unilateral in trigeminal area and is sharp 'stabbing' intermittent, lasting seconds only. Often there is a trigger zone. Typically responds to carbamazepine. No other neurological symptoms or signs.

Investigations/ Diagnosis

Exclude other causes of orofacial pain—local causes (usually dental); neurological disorders (multiple sclerosis or brain tumour); vascular causes (migraine, migrainous neuralgia; cranial arteritis); psychological disorders (atypical facial pain, oral dysaesthesias); referred (cardiac) pain.

Treatment

Carbamazepine and/or phenytoin prophylaxis; cryosurgery to peripheral nerve (rarely, neurosurgery).

Sensory loss in trigeminal region

Causes include: trauma, osteomyelitis, connective tissue disease, drugs and malignant disease.

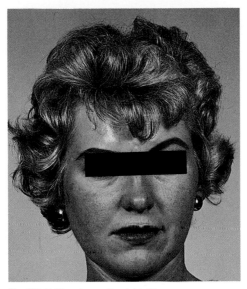

Fig. 162 Bell's palsy on the right side.

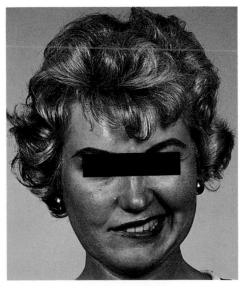

Fig. 163 Bell's palsy: patient smiling.

Ectodermal dysplasia

Incidence/ Aetiology

Rare genetic defect; many variants.

Clinical features

Hypodontia or, rarely, anodontia. Eruption of teeth is delayed. Teeth have a simple conical shape (Fig. 164), and there is frontal bossing and depressed nasal bridge. Hair, eyelashes and eyebrows are sparse and blond. There is an inability to sweat, and nails may be spoon-shaped.

Investigations/ Diagnosis

Clinical features; sweat test occasionally; radiography. Differentiate from chondroectodermal dysplasia (as above plus polydactyly and often congenital heart disease) and other rare syndromes.

Treatment

Restorative care as appropriate.

Cleidocranial dysplasia

Incidence/ Aetiology

Rare. Autosomal dominant condition or mutation.

Clinical features

Exaggerated transverse diameter of cranium with hypertelorism; delayed fontanelle closure; multiple wormian bones; frontal and parietal bossing; depressed nasal bridge; maxillary hypoplasia; underdeveloped paranasal sinuses; high arched palate ($\pm$cleft); tooth eruption delayed or failed; multiple supernumerary teeth; dentigerous cysts; sometimes, hypoplastic enamel (Fig. 165); aplastic or hypoplastic clavicles (shoulders approximate); short stature other skeletal anomalies.

Investigations/ Diagnosis

Clinical features; family history; jaw, skull and skeletal radiographs.

Treatment

Leave unerupted teeth unless complications; orthognathic surgery if necessary.

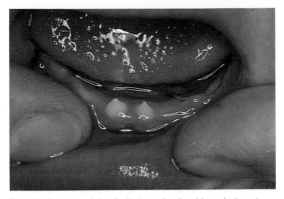

Fig. 164 Ectodermal dysplasia: hypodontia with conical teeth.

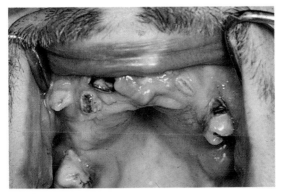

Fig. 165 Cleidocranial dysplasia.

Enamel hypoplasia

Aetiology

Congenital
- Amelogenesis imperfecta (see p. 153).
- Cleidocranial dysplasia (see p. 149).
- Epidermolysis bullosa (see p. 53).
- Vitamin D resistant rickets (hypophosphataemia).
- Congenital hypoparathyroidism, Down and other syndromes.
- Intrauterine infections (rubella; syphilis).

Acquired
- Trauma or infection of developing teeth.
- Prematurity.
- Kernicterus (neonatal hyperbilirubinaemia).
- Neonatal hypoxia or hypocalcaemia.
- Radiotherapy involving developing dentition.
- In early childhood: severe infections, cytotoxic chemotherapy; endocrinopathies (especially hypoparathyroidism) and severe nutritional deficiencies (as in coeliac disease).
- Nephrotic syndrome.
- Severe fluorosis (see p. 153).

Clinical features

Hypoplasia of single teeth   (Turner tooth): usually disturbed odontogenesis caused by periapical infection of deciduous predecessor. It affects premolars mainly, especially mandibular. The crown is opaque, yellow-brown and hypoplastic.

Hypoplasia of multiple teeth: pitting hypoplasia or ring hypoplasia affects part of developing crown. Since systemic disturbances are especially common during the first year of life, defects usually affect tips of permanent incisors and canines (Fig. 166). Congenital syphilis is now a rare cause of hypoplastic notched 'screwdriver-shaped' incisors (Fig. 167; see also p. 39).

Investigations/ Diagnosis

Relevant to possible aetiology. See above.

Treatment

Restorative care as appropriate.

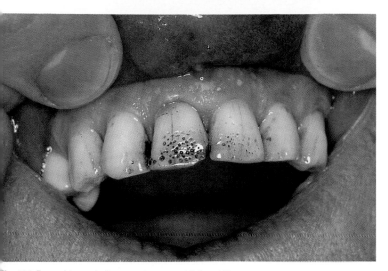

Fig. 166 Enamel hypoplasia secondary to a childhood illness.

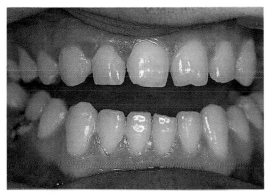

Fig. 167 Syphilis: congenital syphilis showing anterior open bite with peg-shaped incisors.

Amelogenesis imperfecta

*Incidence/
Aetiology*

Uncommon genetic defect with wide variety of
patterns.

Clinical features

Hypocalcified type: normal enamel matrix and
morphology but incomplete calcification. Enamel is
opaque, white to brownish-yellow but darkens with
age. Morphology is normal but the teeth are soft
and chip under attrition.

Hypoplastic type: defective matrix but normal
calcification. Enamel is hard and shiny but
malformed, often pitted and stained (Fig. 168).

*Investigations/
Diagnosis*

Clinical features; family history; radiography of
teeth. Differentiate from fluorosis, tetracycline
staining, dentinogenesis imperfecta, oculo-dento-
digital dysplasia.

Treatment

Restorative dental care.

Fluorosis

*Incidence/
Aetiology*

Particularly common in parts of Middle East, India
and Africa caused by high levels of fluoride in
drinking water. Mild fluorosis may be seen in the
developed world from overexposure to fluoride
from supplements and/or drinking water.

Clinical features

Fluorosis affects many or all teeth.
- *Mildest form*: white flecks or spotting or diffuse
  cloudiness.
- *More severe*: yellow-brown lines or patches.
- *Most severe*: yellow-brown or darker patches,
  sometimes with pitting (Fig. 169).

*Investigations/
Diagnosis*

Data about fluoride content of drinking water.
Differentiate from amelogenesis imperfecta and
tetracycline staining.

Treatment

Veneers or crowns.

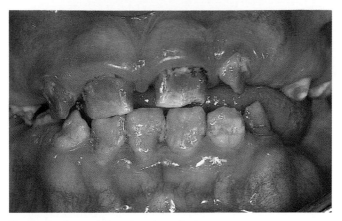

Fig. 168 Amelogenesis imperfecta: hypoplastic type.

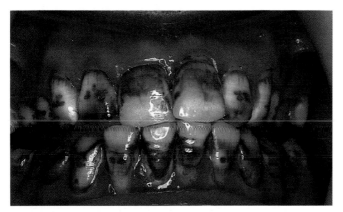

Fig. 169 Fluorosis (severe).

Dentinogenesis imperfecta

Incidence/ Aetiology

Uncommon autosomal dominant condition.

Clinical features

Teeth are abnormally translucent, yellow to blue-grey. Enamel splits off (Figs 170 & 171). Roots are short; pulp is rapidly obliterated by dentine.
- *Type I* (associated with osteogenesis imperfecta): most severe in deciduous dentition; bone fractures; blue sclerae; progressive deafness.
- *Type II* (hereditary opalescent dentine): defect equal in both dentitions.
- *Type III* (Brandywine): associated with occasional shell teeth.

Investigations/ Diagnosis

Clinical features; family history; radiography of teeth/bones.
    Differentiate mainly from amelogenesis imperfecta, tetracycline staining and dentine dysplasia.

Treatment

Restorative dental care.

Tetracycline staining

Incidence/ Aetiology

Should be rare but is still not uncommon where tetracyclines have been given to children or pregnant mothers.

Clinical features

Yellow, brown or greyish pigmentation, especially cervically in anterior teeth (Fig. 172). Teeth may occasionally also be hypoplastic—probably because of the infection for which the drug was used.

Investigations/ Diagnosis

Clinical features; history of exposure to tetracycline. Teeth fluoresce in ultraviolet light if severe. Differentiate mainly from dentinogenesis imperfecta and amelogenesis imperfecta.

Treatment

If causing aesthetic concern: bleaching, veneers or crowns.

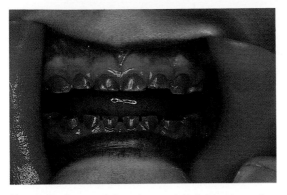

Fig. 170 Dentinogenesis imperfecta: typical discoloration and wearing down of teeth.

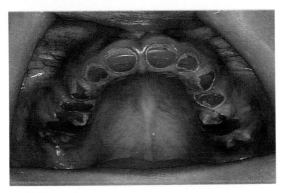

Fig. 171 Dentinogenesis imperfecta: severe attrition in a 14 year old. Pulp chambers are obliterated.

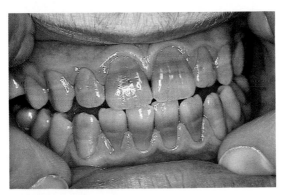

Fig. 172 Tetracycline staining.

Erosion

Uncommon. Repeated and prolonged exposure to acidic solutions (drinks such as carbonated beverages or acidic atmosphere, e.g. chromic or sulphuric acid) or gastric contents (pyloric stenosis, alcoholism or bulimia).

Clinical features
Ingestion of acidic materials produces smooth depressions on labial surfaces of anterior teeth. In regurgitation, palatal and lingual, and sometimes occlusal surfaces are eroded (Fig. 173).

Investigations/ Diagnosis
Careful history and examination. Differentiate from abrasion, dentinogenesis imperfecta and amelogenesis imperfecta.

Treatment
Prevent habit or treat regurgitation. If aesthetically unacceptable, restore.

Abrasion

Incidence/ Aetiology
Common: worsens with increasing age. Usually, caused by vigorous toothbrushing, especially horizontally with abrasive dentifrices.

Clinical features
Initially gingival recession labially and neck of tooth exposed, sometimes with hypersensitivity. Groove forms as cementum and dentine is abraded, especially on canines. Abrasion, if extreme, causes teeth to snap off (Fig. 174). Pulp rarely exposed since reactionary dentine is deposited.

Investigations/ Diagnosis
Careful history and examination.

Treatment
If aesthetically displeasing or causing hypersensitivity, restore with composites.

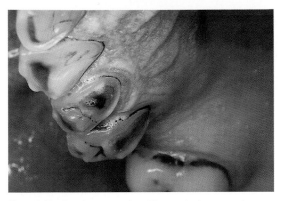

Fig. 173 Erosion due to gastric acid regurgitation secondary to pyloric stenosis.

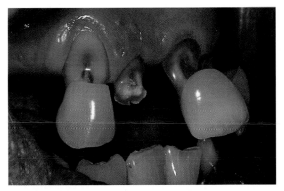

Fig. 174 Abrasion: toothbrushing has abraded teeth but not gingiva.

Classification

Oral lesions in HIV disease have been classified as follows:

Group I
Lesions strongly associated with HIV infection:
- Candidosis
  — Erythematous (see pp. 11 & 77; Fig. 175)
  — Hyperplastic (see p. 67)
  — Thrush (see pp. 63 & 67; Fig. 179, p. 161)
- Hairy leukoplakia (EBV) (see pp. 63 & 67; Fig. 180, p. 161)
- HIV-gingivitis (Fig. 176)
- Necrotizing ulcerative gingivitis (see pp. 37 & 131; Fig. 177)
- HIV-periodontitis
- Kaposi's sarcoma (see p. 79)
- Non-Hodgkin's lymphoma (see p. 45).

Group II
Lesions less commonly associated with HIV infection:
- Atypical ulceration (oropharyngeal) (see p. 25)
- Idiopathic thrombocytopenic purpura (see p. 81)
- Salivary gland diseases
  — Dry mouth
  — Unilateral or bilateral swelling of major salivary glands (Fig. 178)
- Viral infections (other than EBV)
  — Cytomegalovirus
  — Herpes simplex virus (see p. 1)
  — Human papillomavirus (warty-like lesions) (see p. 95): condyloma acuminatum, focal epithelial hyperplasia and verruca vulgaris.
  — Varicella-zoster virus: herpes zoster (see p. 131) and varicella
- Deep mycoses.

Group III
Lesions possibly associated with HIV infection. These are a miscellany of rare diseases.

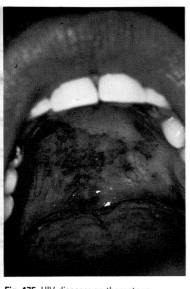

Fig. 175 HIV disease: erythematous candidosis.

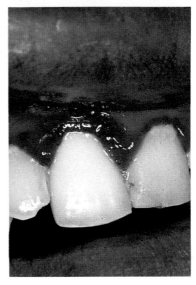

Fig. 176 HIV disease: linear gingivitis.

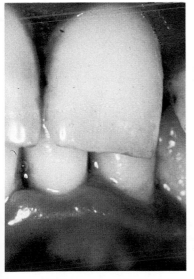

Fig. 177 HIV disease: necrotizing ulcerative gingivitis.

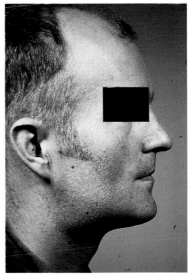

Fig. 178 HIV disease: swelling of submandibular salivary glands.

Oral lesions are common in patients infected with human immunodeficiency virus (HIV) and acquired immunodeficiency syndrome (AIDS), are often the presenting feature, are seen mainly when the CD4 lymphocyte count is low, and may herald deterioration in general health and a poor prognosis. A wide range of oral lesions can be seen, notably fungal and viral infections. However, a panoply of less common lesions can also be seen.

Most HIV infected patients have head and neck manifestations at some stage and oral lesions are often fairly early signs. Pharyngitis, ulcers and cervical lymph node enlargement are fairly common features of primary HIV infection, sometimes with candidosis.

Lymph node enlargement, candidosis (Fig. 179) and hairy leukoplakia (Fig. 180) are most common. All lesions are most likely to occur when the CD4 lymphocyte count falls. Candidosis, hairy leukoplakia and Kaposi's sarcoma are typically associated with CD4 counts lower than 200/cells/mm^3. Major aphthous ulcers and necrotising ulcerative periodontitis almost invariably indicate a CD4 count below this level.

Treatment

Prevention and the treatment of oral disease, particularly painful conditions and opportunistic infections, is especially important in HIV infected persons, in order to maintain quality of life and possibly prevent more serious complications.

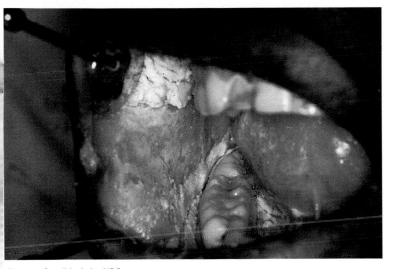

Fig. 179 Candidosis in AIDS.

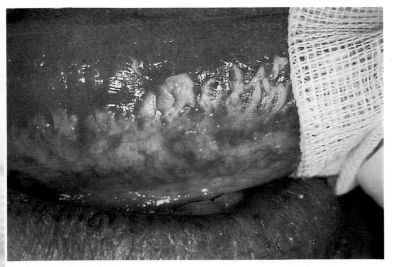

Fig. 180 Hairy leukoplakia.

Appendix: Common treatment measures

Doses given are for fit adults and may need to be modified for other patients. Check pharmacopoiea for other contraindications, cautions and interactions.

Analgesics

Analgesic	Dosage	Contraindications
Non-steroidal anti-inflammatory drugs (NSAIDS)		
Mefenamic acid	250–500 mg up to 3 times a day	Asthma, gastrointestinal, renal and liver disease, pregnancy
Diflunisal	250–500 mg 2 times a day	Pregnancy, peptic ulcer, allergies, renal and liver disease
Non-NSAIDS		
Paracetamol	500–1000 mg up to 6 times a day (max 4 mg daily)	Liver or renal disease or those on zidovudine
Nefopam	30–60 mg up to 3 times a day	Convulsive disorders, pregnancy, elderly, renal, liver disease
Opioids		
Codeine	10–60 mg up to 6 times a day (or 30 mg IM)	Late pregnancy and liver disease
Dihydrocodeine	30 mg up to 4 times a day (or 50 mg IM)	Children, hypothyroidism, asthma, renal disease

Anxiolytics

Anxiolytic	Dose	Comments
Diazepam	2–30 mg daily in divided doses	Avoid in glaucoma Use with caution in the elderly
Temazepam	5–10 mg nocte	Avoid in glaucoma Use with caution in the elderly

Corticosteroids

Corticosteroid	Topical dosage every 6 h	Comments
Hydrocortisone hemisuccinate pellets	2.5 mg dissolved in mouth close to ulcers	Use at an early stage of ulceration
Triamcinolone acetonide in carmellose gelatin paste	Apply to lesions	Adheres best to dry mucosa; affords mechanical protection; of little benefit on tongue or palate
Betamethasone phosphate tablets	0.5 mg; use as mouthwash	More potent than preparations above; may produce adrenal suppression
Beclomethasone spray	1 puff 100 micrograms	"
Budesonide spray	1 puff 100 micrograms	"
Fluocinolone	Apply to lesion	"
Fluocinonide cream, gel or ointment	Apply to lesion	"
Clobetasol cream	Apply to lesion	"
Prednisolone mouthwash	5 mg	"

Systemic immunosuppressants and immunomodulatory agents

Drug	Systemic dose	Comments
Prednisolone	Intially 40–80 mg orally daily in divided doses, reducing as soon as possible to 10 mg daily (give as enteric coated prednisolone with meals)	Limit dosage in hypertension and diabetes mellitus
Azathioprine	2–2.5 mg/kg daily	Contraindicated in pregnancy
Colchicine	500 micrograms, 3 times daily	Contraindicated in pregnancy, elderly, cardiac, renal or hepatic disease
Dapsone	1 mg/kg/day	Contraindicated in G6PD deficiency, pregnancy, cardiorespiratory disease. Monitor reticulocyte count closely
Pentoxifylline	400 mg 2 times daily	Contraindicated in cerebrovascular haemorrhage, myocardial infarction

Antifungals

Antifungal	Dosage and duration (continue for at least 48h after lesions have cleared)*	Possible drug interactions and contraindications
Amphotericin (topical)	10 mg lozenge 100 mg/ml suspension 10–400 mg every 6h for at least 14–21 days	Topical use; no problems
Nystatin (topical)	500 000 unit lozenge 100 000 unit pastille 100 000 unit per ml of suspension 100 000 units every 6h for at least 14–21 days	Topical use; often no problems but unpleasant taste, nausea or gastric disturbance
Miconazole (topical)	250 mg tablet 25 mg/ml gel 250 mg every 6h for at least 14–21 days 50 mg/g denture lacquer; apply weekly for at least 2 weeks	May interact with many drugs including antidiabetics, anticoagulants, phenytoin midazolam, cyclosporin, cisapride and astemizole. Avoid in pregnancy, porphyria. Even topical agent may be absorbed systemically May impair oral contraceptive
Ketoconazole (oral)	200–400 mg daily for at least 14 days	Not absorbed in achlorhydria. May interact with many drugs including anticoagulants, phenytoin, midazolam, cyclosporin, cisapride, zidovudine, terfendine and astemizole. Avoid in pregnancy, porphyria. Hepatotoxic. Expensive. May impair oral contraceptive
Fluconazole (oral)	50–200 mg daily for at least 14 days	May interact with many drugs in antidiabetics, anticoagulants, phenytoin, midazolam, cyclosporin, zidovudine, terfenadine, cisapride and astemizole. Avoid in pregnancy, porphyria. May sometimes be hepatotoxic and myelosuppressive. Expensive

Antifungal	Dosage and duration (continue for at least 48h after lesions have cleared)*	Possible drug interactions and contraindications
Itraconazole (oral)	100 mg capsules 100–200 mg daily for at least 14 days 10 mg/ml liquid 10 ml times daily for at least 14 days	May impair oral contraceptive Not absorbed in achlorhydria. May interact with many drugs including digoxin, sertindole, anticoagulants, phenytoin, midazolam, cyclosporin, simvastatin, terfenadine, cisapride and astemizole. Avoid in pregnancy, porphyria. May impair oral contraceptive

*the higher doses are used in AIDS/HIV infection

Antivirals

Disorder	Drug/dosage
Herpes simplex stomatitis	Aciclovir 100–200 mg tablets 5 times daily, or oral suspension (200 mg/5 ml) 5 times daily
Recurrent herpes	Penciclovir 1% cream every 2h or 5% aciclovir cream every 2h
Herpes varicella-zoster	Aciclovir 800 mg oral 5 times daily or famciclovir 250 mg 3 times daily, or famciclovir 750 mg once daily

(Aciclovir (systemic preparations): caution in renal disease and pregnancy. Occasional rise in liver enzymes and urea, rashes, CNS effects. Famciclovir: caution in renal disease and pregnancy. Occasionally causes nausea and headache.)

Some antidepressants

Antidepressant	Dose	Comments
Amitriptyline	25–75 mg daily divided dose	Contraindicated in recent myocardial infarction, arrhythmias, liver disease
Dothiepin	25 mg 3 times a day or 75 mg at night	Contraindicated in recent myocardial infarction, arrhythmias, liver disease
Clomipramine	10–100 mg daily in divided doses	Contraindicated in recent myocardial infarction, arrhythmias, liver disease
Fluoxetine	20 mg daily	Caution with epilepsy, pregnancy, cardiac, liver, kidney disease, allergy or mania

Index